Praise for *Learnir*

"A truly different approach to smoking cessation.
I could not put this book down."
E. Reynolds, LibraryThing

"Expert authors, encouraging tone, motivational success stories, a
bevy of resources ... **the bible for quitting smoking**."
Bestsellers World

"Shockingly personal and relatable."
Booktopia

"An eye-opening and mind-altering call to take back your power."
Lisa Brown Gilbert, Professional Book Reviewer

"Find reassurance and comfort within the pages of *Learning to
Quit*. It's **exceptional guidance** and support throughout the
entire process earns this book its rating. You'll be glad you picked
up a copy and took the early steps to quitting smoking."
San Francisco Book Review

"Personal stories—told in former smokers' own words—set this
book apart from other guides to quitting smoking."
Kirkus Reviews

"**Powerful book** that will jump start a person's desire to rid
themselves of cigarette smoking and reclaim their power."
Brian Aird, Goodreads

"Sound strategies and guidance that is easy to follow."
J. Armstrong, Amazon

"This book is an unquestionable requirement have for anybody
pondering or resolved to stop [smoking]."
Her Campus Magazine

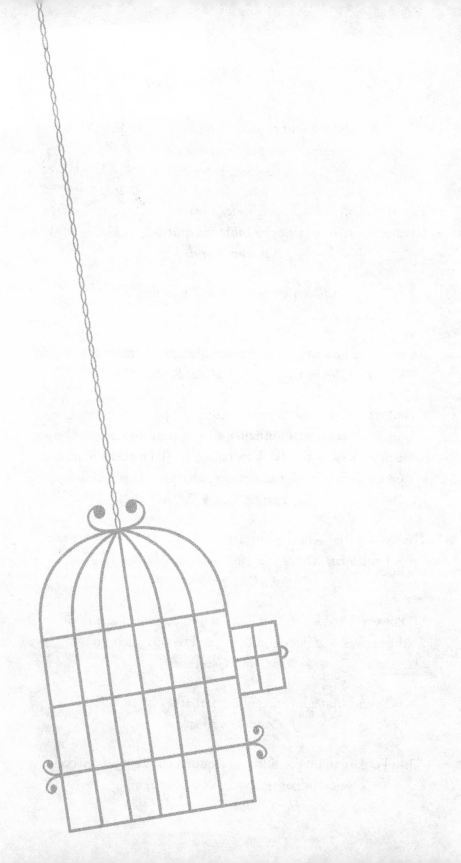

LEARNING to
QUIT

HOW TO STOP
SMOKING
*AND LIVE FREE OF
NICOTINE ADDICTION*

Suzanne Harris, RN, NCTTP
& **Paul Brunetta**, MD

Avasta Press

First published in 2018.
This second edition paperback published 2020 by Avasta Press.
www.AvastaPress.com
Seattle, Washington, United States of America

Copyright © 2020 Suzanne Harris, RN, CTTS, NCTTP and Paul Brunetta, MD
Photos © 2020 John Harding, except where otherwise indicated
Illustrations © 2020 Tess Marhofer, except where otherwise indicated

Book Design by Kelsye Nelson of Avasta Press.
Cover Design by Leonard Buleu.

Ordering information: Quantity sales. Special discounts are available on quantity purchases by corporations, associations, and others. For details, contact the copyright holders at contact@learningtoquit.com, or visit www.learningtoquit.com/order.

PAPERBACK ISBN-13: 978-1-944473-02-0
EBOOK ISBN: 978-1-944473-01-3

Visit www.learningtoquit.com for more
information and free smoking cessation resources.

Dedicated to Clarence Brown - for his inspiration and dedication to people wanting to live a healthier life.

Table of Contents

CHAPTER 9: Changing how we think and what we do: tips and skills to become a non-smoker

CHAPTER 10: Your time is now: gathering resources and successfully stopping smoking

PART TWO Information That Can Support Your Quit Plan

Contents. 285

CHAPTER 11: Tobacco and Lung Disease

CHAPTER 12: Smoking and Cardiovascular Health

CHAPTER 13: Smoking and Cancer Risk

CHAPTER 14: Nicotine and Your Brain

CHAPTER 15: Medications and How They're Used in Smoking Cessation

Ready to start?

🕊 **Jump forward to chapters 9 and 10 when you want to create your quit smoking plan.** Flip back to the personal stories and question exercises whenever you'd like.

🕊 Download the quit plan template, nicotine dependence test and many other free resources listed in this book by visiting:

www.learningtoquit.com**/resources**

Preface

Suzanne in Her Own Words

I am a former smoker and a longtime nurse. I started smoking when I was a teenager, and I thought it was cool and grown-up. If I was in a socially awkward situation, like standing alone at a party, I would light up to give the impression that I was not actually alone and unpopular, but, instead, just taking a cigarette break. For years, I told myself I could quit whenever I wanted. I was well into my twenties before I tried to stop the first time. After that, I tried so many times that I lost count. For some of those years, I worked on a cancer unit, so I had plenty of opportunity to see firsthand some of the most dreadful consequences of using tobacco. Yet I still kept smoking. Finally, I took a deep and honest look at what kept me from succeeding and worked out a real quit plan. Once I got through the hard part of stopping, I was relieved and happy to be smoke-free.

In 1984, I joined the staff of the San Francisco General Hospital Adult Outpatient Medical and Chest Clinics. Many of the patients there suffered from smoking-related diseases, and I was moved to create a program to help them stop. Working with smokers in that setting taught me a lot, and for 24 years I offered six- to eight-week stop-smoking programs and weekly relapse-prevention support groups ("Groups" for short) that helped hundreds of patients become smoke-free. I was also involved in training doctors and nurses how to guide and support patients to stop smoking. In my many years of being in medical settings working with smokers who either want or feel forced to quit, I never met a smoker who was proud of his or her habit—defensive, yes; helpless and even hopeless, yes—but never proud. The last time I felt proud of my smoking was when I was a teenager and first getting hooked.

For most of us, stopping smoking is very hard, perhaps even the hardest thing we've ever done. Some of us tell ourselves that we really like smoking, and that we don't want to stop, effectively covering up a fear that if we tried, we couldn't do it. On the other hand, many smokers who have stopped will say, "Had I known it wasn't going to be so bad, I would have done it a long time ago." Once smokers have gotten through the most uncomfortable parts of becoming a non-smoker, none of them was sorry to have quit.

One of the people who taught me the most about stopping smoking and inspired me to write this book was Clarence Brown (Chapter Eight). As his primary care nurse in the Adult Outpatient Medical Clinic and the nurse in charge of the Chest Clinic, I oversaw Clarence's care. Trying to guide him to better health habits was about as easy as herding cats. And if you lined up a group of smokers and took bets on who would successfully quit, Clarence would not be one of those you would pick. His life was out of control, he smoked and drank a lot, and he used other drugs. Yet even against heavy odds, over a period of seven years, Clarence kept picking himself up from one failed attempt after another until he got himself to a smoke-free life.

More than just about anyone, Clarence taught me that stopping smoking is like learning how to walk: you keep picking yourself up to try again, and no person is a hopeless case. By the time we learn to walk as toddlers, we have spent months developing complex muscle and nervous system control in preparation for our first step. We would have failed in this early challenge if after a few falls we decided it was just too hard and chose to sit down for the rest of our lives. Stopping smoking requires the same persistence, trusting that our misses are what give us the practice and information that we need to make our goal. This is what Clarence did, as you will discover when you read his story.

Being a Certified Tobacco Treatment Specialist (CTTS) has been the most rewarding work in my nursing career. I like knowing that I'm supporting people to do the most important thing they'll ever do for their health and the health of the people they love. Because smoking touches so many parts of a smoker's life, in the process of quitting, people often experience meaningful insights and share intimate experiences. Over and over, I've witnessed former smokers surprise themselves when they became successful and then wondered, "If I can do something as hard as stopping smoking, what else might I be able to do?"

Facing what keeps a smoking habit going means we have to get more honest and direct with ourselves; we not only learn new skills but also learn more about who we really are. So while this is a book about becoming smoke-free, it is also about change; it's about people who have radically changed their lives by ending one huge relationship, their tobacco dependence.

Just imagine: you take smoking out of your daily activities and a space opens up for all kinds of vital things to move in. Joe B. comes to mind. A middle-aged software engineer who spent most of his downtime sitting on the couch eating junk food and watching TV, Joe was nervous when he first joined Group. Actually, he hadn't even decided that he really wanted to quit. But by being open to new ideas and willing to explore his relationship with cigarettes and taking one step at a time, he successfully stopped smoking. Then, to manage anxiety and other withdrawal symptoms, Joe started an exercise program. Within a few weeks, he was walking eight to ten miles up and down the California coast. Next thing, Joe bought himself a camera and began hiking up mountains and taking photographs. In less than a year, he had collected thousands of beautiful images, lost weight, gotten a new hobby, and felt like a new person—because he was a new person. The story of Joe, like that of Clarence, is why I wanted to write this book.

I had been working at San Francisco General Hospital for about ten years when a woman from Group introduced me to John Harding, the photographer for this book. John volunteered to take a photographic portrait for an informational poster for the stop-smoking program, and Clarence Brown volunteered to be the subject. The encounter between the two men was so inspiring that John suggested that he and I work together to collect the stories and portraits of successful quitters.

The third member of our team is Dr. Paul Brunetta. He and I became friends working together in the Chest Clinic at San Francisco General Hospital. Paul's focus was on finding lung cancer and treating it early, and we were both deeply concerned about the tobacco epidemic and the toll it was taking on the lives of our patients. Paul visited some of my Groups and was excited to see what a difference professional support could make for our patients. He recognized how important it is to have stop-smoking classes in medical settings, so when he was appointed an assistant clinical professor at the University of California, San Francisco Medical Center (UCSF), he invited me to join him. Together, we founded the UCSF Tobacco Education Center (TEC) in 1999. We developed a stop-smoking program that meets for two hours weekly for four weeks. Sessions cover issues related to smoking or health, information about medications (presented by a pharmacist), addiction and the brain, and tools for building motivation. All graduates of the program are eligible to attend the weekly Freedom from Smoking Support Group, whether or not they are smoke-free.

Many of these successful quitters are people who have been inspired by the stories in this book and by the stories they have shared with one another. One of them, Jeanne Fontana, came into the TEC for treatment in 2007. She was 61 years old and had developed smoking-related diseases that required her to carry an oxygen tank. At the time, she had many quit attempts behind her, including two stays at a treatment center for smokers, and held little hope that our program would be any better for her than the others.

Jeanne responded well to our friendly, non-fear-based approach, and, somewhat to her surprise, she became smoke-free by the end of the four-week program. She discovered that finding the medication that suited her needs and learning how to support herself in the process were key to her success. Following completion of the program, she regularly attended the Freedom from Smoking Support Group, including when she was in a period of relapse. During that setback, Jeanne struggled with old feelings of hopelessness and helplessness until she learned more about Clarence Brown's own story and used it as a way to take authority over her own.

When Jeanne finally stopped smoking, her quality of life improved, both physically and emotionally. In gratitude for her success, Jeanne made a sizable gift to the TEC with instructions for how her gift should be used: "My desire is to have the program continue to provide the help that I received to as many people as possible." Jeanne understood that tobacco dependence is an incredibly powerful addiction. Identifying with Clarence Brown helped her to persevere in her effort to stop. Now, thanks to her generosity, the lives of hundreds of smokers who pass through the program can be saved. In her honor, the center was renamed the UCSF Fontana Tobacco Treatment Center (FTTC). The FTTC is the fourth member of our team and the most important—it's where stories are told and lives are changed. In reading this book and documenting your own journey, you too will be a part of this community.

Paul in His Own Words

My first cigarette at age nine was such a powerful experience that I can still clearly remember it decades later. For kids, watching adults smoke creates a certain fascination with cigarettes and sends a strong signal that it's what adults do. I remember Marlboro Man billboards and other positive images of smokers that were reinforced through TV and print advertising and movies in the 1970s as I grew up. In high school, I looked forward to smoking at beer-filled weekend parties. It strengthened a bond with one of my best friends, Brian, as something we shared that our other friends didn't. Later, when Brian developed cancer in his early twenties and had surgery and hair loss from chemotherapy, I was with him, taking cigarette breaks as he dragged his IV pole outside Memorial Sloan Kettering Cancer Center. He had to quit smoking, and so did I, and I was going to help him somehow. It taught me how incredibly powerful nicotine addiction is, and it started a lifelong commitment to understanding it.

We both managed to quit, but it wasn't easy and took many, many attempts. Later, in medical school, I began to understand that smoking and tobacco-related disease affect every organ system in the body. In fact, you can learn a tremendous amount about medicine by understanding the effects of smoking on human physiology. This is a modern twist on the famous quote by Sir William Osler from the early 1900s, "He who knows syphilis knows medicine." But it turns out that tobacco-related diseases in the late twentieth century were dramatically more deadly and much more common. Cigarettes kill half of all long-term users—enough to fill three jumbo jets every day of the year. More than 100 million people are estimated to have died from tobacco-related disease in the twentieth century, and we're on track to see approximately one billion premature deaths globally from tobacco in the 21st century.

In my Pulmonary and Critical Care Fellowship at UCSF, I came across a kindred spirit in an amazingly talented and dedicated nurse named Suzanne Harris. Suzanne and I worked together in the Chest Clinic at San Francisco General Hospital, and, together, we cared for a constant stream of patients with tobacco-related COPD and heart disease and lung cancer. This was mirrored in my rotations through the VA hospital where I took care of great veterans who had survived battles for our country but were sickened by long-term tobacco use. Suzanne ran a Group at SFGH, and I asked to sit in. It was one of those moments when you realize you're in the presence of a master doing something very difficult but making it seem effortless. As a former smoker, Suzanne was uniquely able to connect with people in Group with such profound and nonjudgmental empathy, but was also able to guide them toward the next step in a quit plan. When I joined the faculty in the Thoracic Oncology Program focused on lung cancer, early detection, and tobacco education, we were able to find some limited funding from the Mt. Zion Health Fund to create the Tobacco Education Center and hire Suzanne part-time. And, years later, in 2009, a fantastic Group participant named Jeannie Fontana generously donated seed money to secure the long-term survival and expansion of the Fontana Tobacco Treatment Center.

During this time, Suzanne and I created a curriculum for Group sessions and looked for resources to motivate and educate smokers. The medication information we provided was supported by Lisa Kroon, PharmD, who is an expert in smoking-cessation medications (and is now the Chair of Clinical Pharmacy at UCSF). Suzanne strongly believed that positive examples of people reaching their goals was the best source of motivation, but I initially thought that medical information was a powerful motivator. If people could only understand how common and devastating heart and lung disease and cancer are, wouldn't that be more motivational? I now know that Suzanne was right. Foc___g on what you fear most can make some people lose confidence and feel emotionally small. The medical information definitely has its place, though, so we've constructed this book to include both motivational accounts and medical information. The health-related information is written for smokers everywhere who may have no basic knowledge of biology or medicine. I hope I've been able to simplify some of these complex issues to make them relatable.

In all the years that Suzanne has held Groups and Relapse-Prevention meetings, we sought to find a great book that matched our needs and that we could highly recommend to people. This would certainly be easier than writing one. We never found it, and instead embarked on the journey of creating one ourselves. In 2002, we sent book proposals with early ideas to multiple publishing companies and generated a pile of rejection letters. There were already books on the market, we were told, but not the kind we knew would be most useful. In 2012, we tried again and received another batch of rejection letters. For these reasons, we've embarked on our own path, knowing it's the right thing to do and not knowing the outcome. Just as our original program was minimally recognized until a smoker with resources came along and valued it, we hope that you or a friend or a family member will value the stories, photos, and information we've put together in these pages.

Please Note: In Part 1 of this book, in addition to the people whose stories you will read, the voice you hear is Suzanne's. Part 2, the part of the book that addresses medical information, is where you will hear from Paul.

Introduction

Being a smoker takes up a lot of time and energy. Before you leave the house, you must be sure you have your cigarettes and matches or lighter. Once you're out in the world, you're faced with the challenge of finding somewhere you can smoke, knowing that the options are shrinking each day as more and more public places, restaurants, private homes, and even some apartment buildings have become off-limits. When you are at work or socializing, you're nearly always thinking, "When can I get out of here and find a place to light up?" And once you return home at the end of the day, you have to be sure you have enough cigarettes to last the night.

Learning to Quit is designed to help you escape this familiar grind. Stories in this book were originally told in the stop-smoking program that began in 1984 at San Francisco General Hospital and in a related program at the Fontana Tobacco Treatment Center (FTTC) at the University of California at San Francisco Medical Center, which has offered tobacco-dependence treatment to smokers since 1999. The road to a smoke-free life presented in the following pages is based on the highly successful program at FTTC.

Built around the personal success stories of former smokers, *Learning to Quit* is organized into chapters that explore eight open ended questions that confront all smokers:

1. What moves you to be a non-smoker?

2. Who would you be without cigarettes?

3. What do you like about smoking?

4. What is your denial story?

5. What keeps you tied to smoking?

6. If you're already sick, what difference does it make if you smoke?

7. Who other than yourself is affected by your smoking and how could they benefit if you stopped?

8. What is your power and how do you choose to use it?

Each chapter begins with an exploration of one of these questions and then introduces former smokers who tell their own stories and explain how they responded positively to the challenges of the question. The chapter concludes with a summary of what has been covered and with exercises tailored to help you explore the question on your own.

In Part 2, you'll find clarifications of medical terms related to the storytellers' health problems, information on the health effects of smoking, and ways to use medications, including real-world usage developed over years of treating tobacco dependence. Part 2 focuses on lung disease, heart disease, and cancer, as these are the most prominent health problems caused by smoking. They are not the only ones, however, so we encourage you to talk to your doctor about impotence, macular degeneration, and other serious diseases with known connections to tobacco dependence.

Stopping smoking is a very personal process. Some people want lots of medical information and explanations. Others get inspiration from true-life stories. This book is structured so that each question builds on the one before it. But it is also possible to jump around according to what attracts your attention. Pick and choose which parts of this book are of use to you, trusting yourself to be drawn to what will be the most meaningful. Keep a pen or pencil nearby so that when exercises are suggested, you can easily document your thoughts. Make notes in the margins and highlight sections that are especially powerful. This book is a tool, so use it like one. After each chapter, take a few moments to review what you have learned and which skills you can incorporate into your own plan.

People who participate in Groups typically benefit from having a place to regularly check in and stay on track. Some participants report not smoking because they wanted to come to Group and still be smoke-free. Others found a role model in Group and looked forward each week to that individual's leadership. Attending every week keeps your focus on the goal you've set for yourself and gives you an environment where you feel you belong and can receive support. Being in a Group also helps you to understand that some of what you are experiencing is because of the disease you're combating—and that others are living through the same thing.

Reading this book can be like joining a group of people like you, people checking out their options for becoming smoke-free. As you interact with Learning to Quit, it becomes a place you can visit to find support and to retrace your progress, much the way people in our programs have used the Group setting. You might not even be a smoker but have concerns about someone who is, and want a better understanding of the disease. If you are a smoker, you may not have made the decision to stop smoking—and that's okay. We've had many people join our programs to explore what it might take to make the leap and decide they want to try. Some of them surprised themselves by becoming smoke-free at the end of four weeks.

Whatever your relationship to smoking, we hope you will find inspiration, motivation, and guidance in these pages and in the courageous stories of people who want *their* experience to make a difference in *your* life.

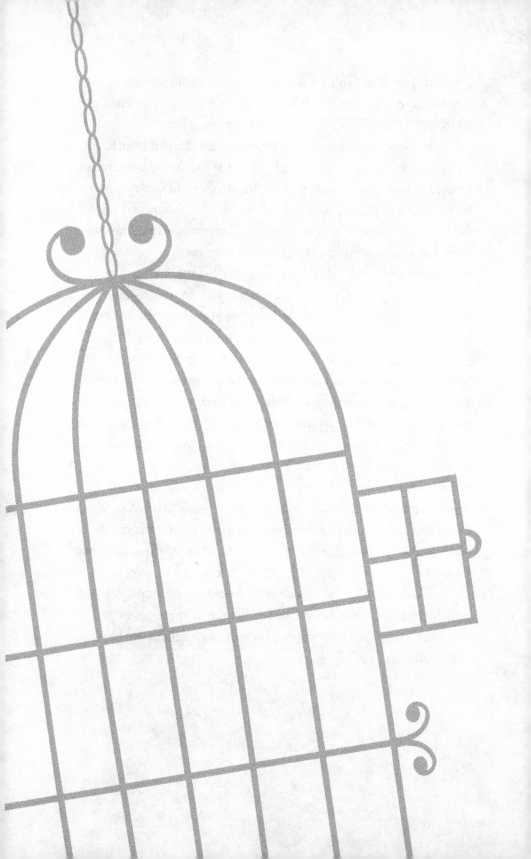

PART ONE

In Their Own Voices

The following eight chapters document relationships Suzanne has had with smokers in her role as a nurse and tobacco treatment specialist. As the people in these stories explored what smoking was for them and what it could mean to become smoke-free, they courageously revealed themselves to her. Their trust, and the journey they took together, enriches her work in deeply satisfying and meaningful ways. She is forever grateful that they were willing to share their stories and process here.

Once you've found your motivation and inspiration from Chapters One through Eight, Chapters Nine and Ten present a concise but powerful guide for your own quitting journey.

CHAPTER ONE

What moves you to be a nonsmoker?

Most smokers are aware of many of the health problems that can come with tobacco use; since 1964 and the first *Surgeon General's Report on Smoking and Health*, we've all been confronted with messages about lung cancer and emphysema, about heart disease and impotence and other health risks associated with smoking. And yet, during years working as a nurse on an inpatient cancer ward, faced with real people enduring surgeries that removed parts of their tongues or jaws, people who were gasping through the final days of lung cancer, I would go on my fifteen-minute break, closet myself in a tiny nurses' lounge, and suck in a couple of cigarettes. I desperately tried to motivate myself with fearful self-talk, but I kept on smoking. My experience showed me that trying to self-motivate with fear or threats is not effective; trying to avoid what we are not supposed to do is much harder than determining what it is that we actually want and going toward that. A powerful inquiry to pursue in the journey to a smoke-free life is to consider what you would like about being a non-smoker. This subtle and powerful shift is a key factor in getting motivated.

> "Trying to avoid what we are not supposed to do is much harder than determining what it is that we actually want and going toward that."

Motivation is the energy to move toward a goal and accomplish it. Motivation may arise spontaneously in response to the perception that things are not how we expect them to be, not how they "should be." When conditions are not what we are comfortable with, we can feel the energy to take action and get things "back to normal." If you want to build motivation to change your behavior, then find ways to take advantage of this energy whenever it arises. Otherwise, the surge will drop off and you will have missed an opportunity to move closer to your goal.

Perhaps this will be an example to which you can relate: imagine you are having some work done to your home. You are in the final stages of completing a remodel that includes repairing walls, painting, and the like. Finally, everything but the finishing touches is complete. The rooms are painted, and the only thing left to be done is to install light plates over the switches. For several days you will notice this last unfinished element and it will nag at you. However, if you let enough time go by, your mind will become accustomed to the view and you will no longer notice the light plates are missing. It could be weeks or months or forever before you finally take care of this last detail. Likewise, if you want to quit smoking, once you become skilled at noticing motivation as it arises, find immediate ways to take action—to do something real. Perhaps join a group (in the real world or online) dedicated to stopping smoking. Using this precious energy will help it to grow and carry you toward your smoke-free goal.

Furthermore, you don't have to passively wait for motivation to arise; you can take an active part in growing your own motivation for change. For starters, let's look at two kinds of motivation: fear-based and desire-based. Smokers are faced with plenty of fear-based motivation. Doctors, nurses, and concerned loved ones may, out of frustration, ignorance, or helplessness, push to convince you to stop, citing fearful consequences if you don't: "Mr. Brown, if you don't stop smoking immediately, you are going to kill yourself." Or, "Mommy, I don't want you to die; please stop smoking." Because smokers tend to medicate anxiety and other difficult feelings with cigarettes, these fearful messages often backfire: the smoker hears the message and immediately wants to smoke. Also, smokers are like anyone else who, when pushed, responds with resistance: "You're not the boss of me. I smoke because I like it and I'll stop whenever I please." Resistance often covers the fear that you cannot quit. Regardless, most of us do not like being told what to do and will react defensively by doing more of what we're being told to stop.

Fear as a motivator restricts behavior. It is all about avoiding one thing and doing something else that we "have to or should do." Who of us wants to do what we have to do, what we should do? When we are in fear, we can feel weak, powerless, hopeless, stuck, and even worthless. Working on a cancer unit where I was faced with daily reminders of the dreadful things that could happen to me if I kept smoking, I felt frightened, and that fear led to more smoking as a means of dealing with the anxiety. And my smoking kept the fear alive, reminding me with every puff about what was disturbing me so deeply.

> "Most of us do not like being told what to do and will react defensively by doing more of what we're being told to stop."

When it comes to changing unhealthy behaviors, it could be that the only positive function for fear is that it snaps us out of denial. If the dentist were to tell you that you need a biopsy of a suspicious area on your tongue, you would likely be shocked out of complacency about smoking. But to persist in beating yourself into change by telling yourself scary stories about what could happen just weakens and undermines you, increasing a feeling of powerlessness and worthlessness. These are not feelings that support successful and enduring behavioral change. In short, use any fear you feel to pull you out of your denial about smoking. Then, move to the next step and start looking at what you can imagine you will enjoy about being smoke-free.

It is this desire-based motivation that can really help get you moving. People naturally move toward what they desire. Like the proverbial donkey, if someone gets behind us to push and bully us along, we dig in our heels; however, we willingly follow the dangling carrot. Desire-based motivation puts us back in control; it encourages action and sets us in motion to achieve. We are doing what we want to do, going after what we want to have. Following your desires builds confidence. We feel strong and empowered and optimistic. Being motivated by desire supports self-esteem and gives us the sense of having options. Most important, it helps create lasting change.

When looking at fear-based motivation and desire-based motivation, remember that it's not just what gets said to you from outside that makes a difference; even more important is what you say all day long inside your own head. Smokers sometimes try to abuse themselves into stopping: "Why am I so stupid? I've got to stop smoking." Without being aware of it, they set up a battle within themselves between the part that says, "I have to" and the part that says, "No, I won't, I don't have to." This split makes it so much more difficult to move forward. It is literally like trying to drive with the brakes on.

It isn't the things that are happening to us that cause us to suffer; it's what we say to ourselves about the things that are happening. The truth you believe and cling to makes you unavailable to hear anything new. **Pema Chödron**

Bill Spangenberg

Knowing how to ask for help is a skill. Bill wasn't pushed to stop smoking until it became a question of survival, and then he recognized he couldn't do it on his own. Once he found the object of his motivation, he sought out a program that could support him. He had started smoking, in part, to become part of a peer group; to stop, he needed a support group of other people working toward the same goal. Interestingly, while Bill felt like a social outsider when he was young, the process of stopping smoking gave him an experience of belonging. The original motivation to smoke never subsided and, ultimately, led him to a healthier satisfaction of his need.

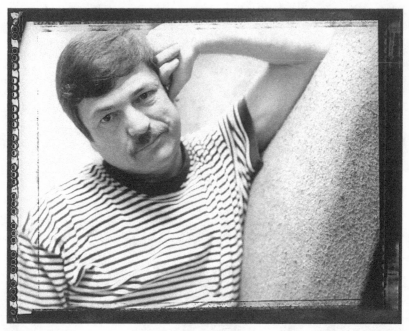

Bill Spangenberg   Photo by John Harding

Bill Spangenberg, in His Own Voice

What I hear out of everybody is, "Smoking is hurting your health, causing cancers, messing up your lungs." I already have a bad disease that is going to kill me. I am less concerned about [getting] cancer than I am about anything else. I look at a billboard that says, "Smoking causes cancer" and I say, "So?" Put something up there that is going to mean something to me. "Smoking costs money." Point blank.

Once a month, I [have] X number of dollars to spend after my bills are paid. How much I had to spend on cigarettes was an expense just like rent, which was nonadjustable. On disability, my income was $926.00. Five cartons cost $125.00 a month. Either I bought groceries or I smoked. Because of the HIV, I could get some other benefit packages, but it was very common for me to go the last two weeks of the month with nothing but cigarettes and a little bit of food. Cigarettes came in front of food. It was major depression, a feeling of being trapped, a feeling of panic.

My father smoked, so we wanted to smoke. I hated it. I picked it up when I was seventeen. In my school district, I was left out; I was not part of anything. When I went to work eight miles away with a whole different group of people, I said, "I am going to be just like they are." They smoked, so there was major peer pressure for me to smoke. What would have made a difference to me at age seventeen is if I had been shown I fit in without smoking. My parents taught me work ethics, but they did not teach me the social thing.

There are a lot of conflicts in smoking. I liked it because it was something I had to myself, but it also isolated me from other people. "Dinner is going to be ready in five minutes; can I hurry up and sneak another cigarette in, or should I wait?" And if you wait, halfway through dinner you want that cigarette that you didn't have earlier. You've got to pat your pockets before you go out, to make sure you have enough to get there and get around and make sure you have a lighter that works. I couldn't go out wearing a t-shirt: t-shirts don't have a pocket in them for cigarettes. That stupid kind of stuff was the bad stuff.

At a pack and a half to two packs a day, I knew I wanted to quit, I knew it was going to be hard, and I wasn't ready. I was not willing to go through the work of quitting. The work was taking an honest open look at myself and getting rid of something that was a detriment, that was the work.

I was afraid to quit because I knew there was no way I could do it by myself. If I could do it by myself, I would have quit a long time ago. Daily, I would get up and say, "I am not going to smoke today," as I reached for them, so I knew it was something I was not going to do by myself.

I don't believe people are at ease asking for help. Human nature says, I ought to be able to do it myself." Anytime anybody reaches out for help, they are taking a chance. We are afraid we are a failure, afraid of rejection, afraid of what other people think of us, afraid we are alone, and that nobody else has the same problem we do. One of the things that really kicked me in the butt was that my dad smoked for twenty years, and one day he got tired of it and put them on top of the refrigerator and forgot them. He has no concept of people not being able to do that.

> "I knew I was going to have to quit soon because my money was running out."

I was tired of being sick and tired. I knew I was going to have to quit soon because my money was running out. I looked at doing it realistically. For me, it was more a chemical habit than anything, so I used the patches. I set up that network of support. I found some experts [who] gave me the information I needed, showed me what steps to take, showed me the work I needed to do.

The smoking-cessation Group was wonderful. I found other people in the same position I was in, and it made me feel good because I was not alone. I met people there who were encouraging and interested in my progress. The Group let me come into it and be part of it. The support taught me to get support and use it. If I get panic-stricken, I use the deep breathing. It helps me to relax and slow down.

The anticipation was more frightening than the actual quitting; the actual stopping was an exercise. I anticipated mood swings, being angry all the time, and eating constantly. That didn't happen. My eating increased, but my moods didn't swing all that much. I kept in my mind, "Oh, it is because I quit smoking; it is going to smooth out in a few days," and it did. Until I quit smoking, I was up at 5:30 in the morning to have a cigarette. Now I sleep until 8:30 or 9almost every day.

> "I look at quitting smoking as getting rid of a bad thing and expanding the good things I already have."

A lot of what I learned in AA I transferred into stop smoking: It is not the second or third cigarette that is going to get you hooked, it is the first one; I didn't quit smoking for the rest of my life, but I quit for today; tomorrow is not here; it doesn't make a difference how long ago you quit; you are only one step away from going back to it.

If I make it a big deal, I am going to go back to smoking. It is a major step in my life, but it is not a big deal. If it is a big deal, it is something that I keep in my mind all the time, like being an alcoholic and working in a liquor store. It is always right there in front of you.

I look at quitting smoking as getting rid of a bad thing and expanding the good things I already have. I spend more time learning things like science. On the internet, they have a lot about space. I am absolutely fascinated with it. I have become more social, my number of friends has increased, the activities that I do increased. I cook more. I didn't bring a new package into my life; I expanded things that I already had.

Two things I would not do: one is pick up a drink, and two is pick up a cigarette. You find other things to do. Smoking was always my backup. When I got upset, if I got confused, I lit up a cigarette and it bought me time. Now, I don't have something I can mechanically use, so mentally I have to slow down. Now I still stop and think, but I just don't go through the light-up-the-cigarette process, and I think more clearly and more rationally.

Common sense says that if you see the inside of a cancerous lung and know it was caused by smoking, you are going to quit. That is the logical way to think; it doesn't work. What works is when somebody runs out of money and realizes they can either eat or smoke. You are put into a corner and you have to make a decision.

Nicotine is the most addictive drug in the world. If you don't make it, keep trying because if you give up, then you have failed. If you keep trying, you are a winner even if you don't make it for a while. I accomplished something really big. I eat well on the same amount of money I used to starve.

What moved Bill to be a nonsmoker?

Bill's conscious motivation was to be able to eat. He didn't have enough money for both food and cigarettes—and because food is a basic survival need, having enough to eat was a positive force for becoming smoke-free. Bill stayed clear on what he would gain by becoming smoke-free, and the object of his motivation provided him with a strong pull forward.

Success is the sum of small efforts, repeated day
in and day out. **Robert Collier**

Yan Spruzina

Yan was born after the Communists took over Czechoslovakia. He
was a young boy when his sister's boyfriend was sent to prison.
At the time, collecting cigarette packages was a way of getting
permission to visit the prison. Smoking was encouraged because
taxes on cigarette packages provided money to the state. In the
process of collecting the packages, Yan began smoking.

Years later, in the United States, he was still smoking. His
habit caused frequent ear infections, and Yan was scared that being
sick and missing work would make him lose his job and be unable
to pay his bills. He knew he had to do something or he could end
up homeless and never be able to get back to Czechoslovakia to
see his family. He also felt a lot of anger at the tobacco industry
and wanted to show that he wouldn't be used for their profit. He
decided to stop smoking.

A heavy smoker, Yan consumed a minimum of sixty
cigarettes a day. Smoking helped him power through his job as
a baker, revving him up to make three hundred pies in a day. He
liked the sense of accomplishment and the accolades he received
for such incredible productivity. He enjoyed the camaraderie of
smoking with co-workers and was concerned about how he'd
replicate that pleasure. But more than the pleasure of smoking, he
wanted freedom, better health, and a better quality of life. In terms
of developing motivation, he understood everybody must find out

"The real enjoyment is without the cigarette."

for themselves what's important for them. He wanted to enjoy life. And, according to Yan, "You don't enjoy the life with a cigarette; you feel more miserable after a minute, you are more tired; so why have it? I don't enjoy the life with a cigarette; believe me, neither do you, you just don't know it yet. The real enjoyment is without the cigarette."

After he had quit smoking and was facing the challenge to remain smoke-free, Yan used his attachment to the Group to keep himself focused: he did not want to let down his friends in the Group. He imagined being accompanied by Group members with whom he felt a connection and who reinforced his desire to keep coming to meetings; there, he was able to report that he was successfully smoke-free. Highly energetic by nature, smoking turned him into a marathon baker. Once he finally stopped, he was happy to report: "I just work like a normal human being. I negotiate my rights or limits. Before stopping smoking, I'd stay up for thirty-six hours straight, baking and smoking."

By becoming smoke-free, Yan reclaimed his autonomy. He was no longer supporting a state or an industry that did not uphold his well-being as valuable. He ensured a greater likelihood of the health he needed to keep working, and he lived more in balance, with reasonable productivity at work.

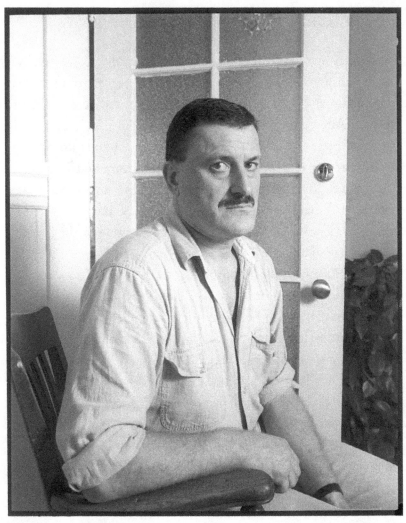

Yan Spruzina   Photo by John Harding

Yan Spruzina, in His Own Voice

I was born in Czechoslovakia after the Second World War. My dad did insurance work for a state-run company; my mom was a housewife and not happy. We were upper middle class before the war. After the Communists took over in 1948, everybody was poor, but we got poorer than poor. I was born into poverty, but my mother remembered how we were before and I missed it through her. My father and my mother didn't smoke before the Communists nationalized our property; they started to smoke after. I was hooked up on cigarettes when I was fifteen. It was a macho thing to do, just like here.

In 1968, with the riots against the Russians, I ran away to Germany. In 1980, I came to the United States from Germany. I started to have wheezing asthma. Then came the California Health Department saying that smoking is bad. I heard more and more negative things, that it is a big addiction, and I started to think about it. When I started to be aware that it is more dangerous than they [the tobacco companies] had led us to believe, I started to look for low-tar and lower-nicotine cigarettes.

I tried to stop by myself, and it was absolutely hopeless. I didn't have enough strength. After half an hour [of] no cigarettes, I went nuts. I was hoping that they would have some brain pills, some easy way to stop smoking with help from outside, rather than from within me. A bad ear infection gave me a real scare. I started to vomit, and I was scared I would lose my job; I wouldn't be able to pay my bills. They said, "It's from cigarettes; you have to stop smoking."

Going to the smoking-cessation classes, it started to pile up; it just became important to be free. I started to be conscious of the daily nuisances: like having to have enough cigarettes to make it through the night, to check if I had three packs to go to work. Once I started to realize the little things and to pile them up, they struck me as being an enormous time waste.

The Group support was a major motivation. The Group became almost a substitute for family. You try to mobilize as much as you can to do good for the whole Group, for yourself. After they put so much work into me, I wanted to give something back. I have a lack of responsibility, but it was there, and it started to grow down on the bottom of my soul.

What else stuck in my head? That we must not consider ourselves as failures and feel guilty, that it's not our fault that we are smokers. The phrase, "It's not your fault that you smoke" just set me free somehow; it was like miracle phrase, one of what I now call the commandments. "It's not your fault," first of all. And: "You want to be free," free to be like others, free from the cigarettes. Then the anger at the tobacco companies: they think we are fools and they fool us; they go against us. Anger was a good force, a positive force, to show them that they cannot do with me as they chose.

> "You must be ready to counter the advertisement in your brain that says it is okay to smoke: "I don't need the cigarette, I'm better than this, enough of the dependency."

When I was ready to quit, I bought apples, carrots, and chewing gum with nicotine. In the morning I went on the buses, but I'm was nervous, so I went on the beach with water and hot, spicy nachos; soy sauce; and Tabasco sauce. I read the notes of what I had learned through the classes, and I started the commandments, repeating them over and over again, from 11 a.m. until sunset. Then I started to have the first feelings of joy that I could breathe better and my nose started to open up. I started to smell the smell of the sea, for the first time in ten years, and then I started to remember to expand my way to the freedom, telling myself that since this was already twenty hours without a cigarette, after thirty years of smoking, it would be a shame to mess up such an achievement.

I was so exhausted I slept ten hours, and then I started to be proud of myself that for the first time in thirty years, I was without a cigarette for twenty-four hours. I went to work, proud, pumping myself full. That kept the craving away. I made it through the pressure at work, still reciting the commandments: "Step to the freedom … better health … better quality of life … more money."

After three years, I could come off taking extra-strength Sudafed for my sinus problem. Not taking the pills, not having the ear infections, nose infections, having more energy, not going home from work extremely exhausted: that's so positive. Simply being able to enjoy going to see friends, going to the movies, which I didn't do for three years because I had smoked myself to exhaustion. It does do good things, this California, pounding on smokers; it annoys you at the beginning; then it does open up your brain to the no-smoking programs.

Even if you don't believe that you will be successful, [the belief you can quit] starts to prevail; it starts to grow in you, and the positiveness starts to be strong. There will be all kinds of little voices bombarding you: "Have another cigarette." Be ready for them. You must be ready to counter the advertisement in your brain that says it is okay to smoke: "I don't need the cigarette, I'm better than this, enough of the dependency." Those are really miracle slogans, which work.

I feel confident, victorious, and proud. I am so strong now I'm passionate about it. *I won't smoke.* I smoked thirty years, and I just don't need the cigarettes. I don't enjoy the life with a cigarette. Believe me, neither do you; you just don't know it yet. You will stop smoking, too. You will realize that the real enjoyment is without the cigarette.

What moved Yan to be a non-smoker?

Yan's motivations were to free himself from the burden of tobacco dependence, to feel physically and emotionally stronger, and to more fully enjoy his life without the fear of what might happen if he made himself sick with smoking. He focused on the positive gains that he understood would be his when he became smoke-free.

May you take time to celebrate the quiet miracles that seek no attention. **John O'Donohue**

Cecilia Brunazzi

Cecilia is a connoisseur of culture and fine living. She is known for her stylish dinner parties and delicious Italian cooking; she also loves going to museums and the theater. When she found herself dealing with frequent respiratory infections, she could no longer ignore the toll smoking was taking on her. Even more motivating than that, she wanted to be free to enjoy the things she loves without the negative effects of having to deal with smoking.

When she began the process of stopping smoking, Cecilia already had several positive practices in place. She had integrated regular daily exercise into her life, walking to as many of her destinations as possible and leaving the car at home. Several times a week, she went to yoga classes and enjoyed swimming, as well. A tiny, intense woman, Cecilia approached her new challenge with the same level of focus and presence with which she lived the rest of her life. Having experienced for years what it was like to be a smoker, she set out to discover what it would be like to live smoke-free.

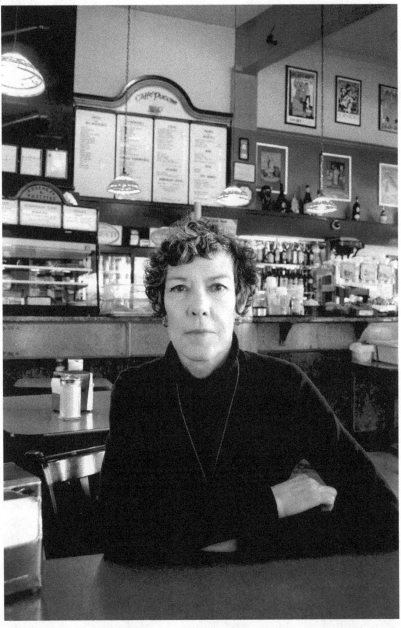

Cecilia Brunazzi   Photo by Cristina Taccone

Cecilia Brunazzi, in Her Own Voice

I started smoking when I went to boarding school. There was a smoking lounge for seniors only; it was a senior privilege and it seemed adult and glamorous. My father was a heavy smoker; he had cigarettes in his breast pocket. I remember as a child sitting on his lap and smelling the tobacco. I was close to my father, so I think those were some of the reasons that I started. Then I went to college in North Carolina, a big tobacco state. Cigarettes were so cheap because there weren't the taxes that there are in other states.

The first time I actually tried to quit was in my twenties. I only quit for about a week. I tried again in my thirties and lasted a little longer. I never quit for a very long stretch of time. I didn't try again until I came to the program. I remember seeing in a newsletter something about the program and thinking, "Okay, maybe I cannot quit smoking, but I can make this call." I called and left a message and then you called me to say the program was beginning, and I went, "Oh, did I sign up for that?" Then that same psychology kicked in, and I thought, "Maybe I can't quit smoking, but at least I can go warm a chair and see what happens." That is how I got myself there.

I made it to a year and that was it. The famous being-on-vacation-and-having-one-after-dinner scenario. The one after dinner lasted for a couple of years. Then I got disgusted with myself and called and asked if I could do the program again; it seemed the right thing to do was to start over from the beginning.

When I was a child, I had severe asthma and allergies, and as an adult, I developed mild asthma again. I came to the Group the first time after I had three bouts of really bad acute bronchitis. All of a sudden, this just started happening to me and it was scary. I had to take very strong antibiotics, and I felt rotten. I had a chronic smoker's cough, and every time I quit smoking, that cough was gone in about two days, and every time I would start smoking, it was back in about two days. I also became acutely aware of the tyranny of being addicted to cigarettes, how much they were controlling me. I remember being invited to someone's house

> "... every time I quit smoking, that cough was gone in about two days, and every time I would start smoking, it was back in about two days."

for dinner, and being completely anxious all the way over to the dinner, thinking, "Is there going to be a place where I can smoke?" I remember wanting but dreading to go to a long performance because I knew I would want a cigarette, and could I sprint outside quickly enough during intermission to suck down two cigarettes and then sprint back in? Smoking was starting to really make me miserable in situations that could be pleasurable; the experience of having to have a cigarette was interfering with other kinds of enjoyment. If I was feeling miserable about myself anyway, when I was smoking cigarettes, that made me feel more miserable, because I thought, "Oh I can't even quit smoking." Everything was just stacking up to help me realize that it wasn't worth it, it was controlling my life and interfering with my enjoyment of things.

When I was smoking in between my two quits, I encountered an acquaintance who was visiting from New Mexico. Since I had last seen her, her multiple sclerosis (MS) had really accelerated and she was in a wheelchair. I said, "I am going outside to have a cigarette." and she looked at me and said, "Oh my goodness, you still smoke? Oh, you poor thing." And I thought, "Here is this woman with MS in a wheelchair, pitying *me*." She didn't say it maliciously; she said it in a very compassionate way. That is all she said, but it was very powerful.

During that same time, my dear friend died of lung cancer. I was one of the caretakers. She only lived eight months from the time she was diagnosed, and I was smoking when she first was diagnosed; during her illness, I stopped for the second time.

During those last two serious attempts, some combination of aerobic exercise had been completely necessary for me. Swimming has been useful because you are so aware of your breath, and yoga has been really useful, both as a physical exercise and because breathing is part of yoga.

I found the Relapse-Prevention Support Group to be really important. The Group is not judgmental if you are smoking; there is a lot of encouragement given to people who are sort of like athletes in training. People don't just go out and run a record two miles; you have to train for it. Quitting smoking is a big challenge, like an athletic challenge, so even though I would try, I would stop a little bit, and I would relapse. Eventually, I got tired of that cycle of trying, relapsing, smoking a while, getting disgusted with it, trying again.

I remember having the thought, "Well, you really know what it is like to smoke, and you are not that happy with it; but you don't know what it is like to not smoke for a long time so that would be kind of interesting." I decided to give it another really strong try; I started going to the Group more consistently. I wanted to quit right before my birthday; symbolically that seemed like a nice thing to do for myself. I remember thinking, "I don't want to quit on the exact day because I don't want it to be a really hard day," so I quit a couple of days before my birthday. All those trial runs were helpful because I could plan better and knew better what to expect, to give myself permission to watch a lot of movies, to just distract myself in the beginning. I used the patch and a little bit of gum, and I actually ended up not being miserable on my birthday.

A former smoker I spoke to many years ago compared the experience of quitting smoking to childbirth: both are extremely painful but as time goes on, you develop this kind of amnesia about how difficult and painful the experience is. That is a kind of slippery slope of smoking that you don't remember just how excruciatingly hard and challenging it is at the beginning. Going to the Group and seeing and hearing people in various phases of the process— some people who are trying to gear up to quit, being unhappy with themselves, making vows, being fearful, all the things I went through—and then hearing people who are in the initial stages, hearing about their experiences, has been a great reminder of how difficult it is. It is a big red flag: *you do not want to have to do this again; it is just not worth it.* Hearing corroborating stories from different people about the "just-one" pitfall, "I am going to have just this one" is so common. You can say it to yourself and sort of ignore it, but if six other people say they have had that experience, you know it is really something that just doesn't work. Also, hearing about how other people deal with situations that could be perilous: vacations; travel; being in another country; sometimes being alone; or thinking, "nobody will know except for me": hearing just how common those things are reinforces what you have to be vigilant about; our addictive parts are insidiously creative.

In my office long ago, they banned smoking inside the office, and I used to smoke in front of the computer and I found out that "Hey, I could still work and not smoke." It is possible to uncouple these things; it takes a while; maybe you are not as efficient at doing that thing without the cigarette, but it really is possible. That is useful to think about, if you are still smoking; think about a situation in which you *used to* be able to smoke. I remember, years ago, smoking in the movies, for heaven's sakes. I think about one of those situations in which one used to smoke and how it was restricted; well, people still go to movies, they still eat in restaurants, do a whole range of things without smoking.

Now, occasionally, if I am in a highly stressful situation, I will think about cigarettes. I do the deep breathing and I try to distract myself. I try not to dwell on the thought, not to indulge the longing. It is possible to train yourself to say, "Okay, I had that thought, and I am not going to think about it." As opposed to, "Oh, gee, a cigarette would be so nice. I wonder what it would taste like." But if you go there, it is making it harder on yourself, and it is just as if you had a puff; it makes it harder on you.

One thing I focus on when I am around smokers is what a short duration the satisfaction has. You smoke a cigarette that you think is going to be so great, and it is over in a minute or two, and then you have got to figure out what to do with the cigarette butt and all that. Now, I look at someone smoking and I say my mantra to myself: "I'm so glad I don't have to do that anymore."

Fight the feeling that if you relapse it is permanent, and that you are a miserable failure because you relapsed. Feeling like you are a failure feeds into not quitting again. Get back on that horse after you have fallen off. Anything that is difficult takes practice, so it is ridiculous to think that you can just quit smoking in a snap; it does require practice because it is challenging.

People shouldn't beat themselves up about relapsing because that is just part of the recovery, and the sooner you can stop feeling bad about it, the sooner you can get your oomph together to try again. And particularly at the beginning, practice that old "one-day-at-a-time" thing. I couldn't even think about *never* smoking again; it was just too scary. Then I got to six months, and I said, "Okay, I am going to see if I can make it to a year." When I got to a year, I said, "Okay, I made it to a year before; I am going to see if I can make it to eighteen months." I don't have to do that goal-setting any more, but for about two years, I really needed to do that.

I smoked for forty years. If I am trying to confront something that I find extremely difficult, I sometimes have the thought, "Well, if I could quit smoking, I could do this."

What moved Cecilia to be a non-smoker?

Smoking interfered with Cecilia's enjoyment of the cultural experiences that define her. Quitting smoking opened her to the freedom of being present with what gives her joy and brings meaning and quality to her life.

Proceed as if success is inevitable. **Unknown**

Mary Adams

Not unlike Cecilia, Mary is a tiny, wiry, powerful woman. Looking decades younger than her actual age, Mary is as devoted to her family as anyone I've known. She deeply loves her children and was tormented by the choices they were making. Both of her adult children were casualties of the San Francisco drug epidemic. Her son was in prison and her daughter was prepared to sell anything to fund her drug habit. Helpless in the face of the calamity of her children's lives, Mary wanted to model for them that it is possible to do something really hard: she decided to stop smoking.

Mary knew there was no way she could make her kids stop using drugs. She understood that we cannot set goals for other people; the only person she can effectively change is herself, so Mary decided to use herself as an example. She lived in a household where everyone smoked except for the babies (who were in effect "smoking" the second-hand smoke of the adults). In addition, no one in the home wanted her to stop, and her husband would go so far as to try to taunt her into having a cigarette: blowing smoke into her face, he'd say, "Come on, I know you want one. Here, here's some smoke just for you." But Mary was undeterred. Her goal had to do with what was most precious to her: a future for her children and grandchildren.

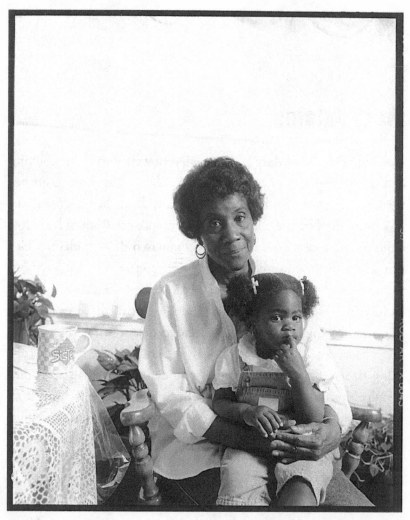

Mary Adams

Photo by John Harding

Mary Adams, in Her Own Voice

We lived in a housing project. I was nine or ten, and I started off smoking Kools. I had some friends that lived in the neighborhood. We were doing something just to be how kids get into things. We would be about five or six of us and have a pack, and we would go into the park, off in the trees, and just smoke, smoke, smoke. At that time, cigarettes were so cheap, and you could buy them without your parents.

My dad was a longshoreman. He would put a cigar in his mouth every now and then but never had it lit. He worked nights and he kept a tight ring on us, everything we did; my daddy was a strict man. When I was a teenager at my dad's house; we had a back room and I didn't realize that the cigarette smoke was going to trail up. That's when I heard him call out: "Who's in there smoking?" I finally said, "Me," and he came with his belt and, boy, he got me good. He did not want us to smoke at all; we were not allowed. We hid it, and we kept on smoking.

My mother, she might have smoked just sometimes, if I remember correctly. My mother died at age twenty-eight, leaving seven children. I was ten. I am the third child. We're all still alive. And we are close when tragedies happen, especially the sisters. My older sister and I we are really close 'cause we kind of think along the same lines. She quit smoking years ago. Just quit. She had a son that had asthma really bad, and he would come over and take the cigarette out of her mouth: "You are not supposed to smoke." She is so happy that I have quit smoking, she don't know what to do.

For years, it was making me feel bad. I felt sluggish. No energy. I was only 98 pounds. My doctors were saying I should quit, 'cause I had high blood pressure. I started getting to the point where I couldn't breathe, walking—I couldn't breathe. When they thought there was something wrong with my esophagus, I knew it was time for me to quit.

I was trying to find a clinic to go to that was affordable and that is how I found out about the stop-smoking program at the hospital. I went through it two or three times. I didn't really stop smoking until I started constantly attending the support Group every Monday.

The hardest thing for me when I quit was not being able to, after I eat, have that cigarette. That was the hardest thing for me. I would get up from the table right away and either wash dishes or fold clothes, or I did something with my hands; and eventually it went away.

When I did quit, I made up my mind that whatever happens nothing was gonna make me smoke again. It was a determination. It was just something in me. I just made up my mind that this was something that I was not going to do anymore. Coming to the support Group encouraged me, and even when I stopped coming regularly, you guys would be on my mind.

My husband, he wanted me to smoke, 'cause he was a smoker and he couldn't quit. He would blow smoke in my face, telling me that I wasn't serious and that I might as well start up and smoke. I told him, "For one thing I am doing this for myself, but I want to show my children that if you really make up your mind you can quit doing something that is bad for you"; and they know that I would really rather smoke than eat.

All the things that have gone on in my life, I could really have gone back to smoking. My kids are drug-users; my son goes back and forth to jail. Drugs really do my kids bad. I've never seen anything like it in all my life. It has devastated my family, it really has. It's just unbelievable. Crack cocaine, if I knew who invented that mess, boy, I think I would want to kill him and go to jail and serve time for it because I think that is the most devastating. I hate it for anybody, but I truly hate for a woman, 'cause they tell me a woman will do anything for that drug and I just hate to think what is happening out there. My two kids, they used to never smoke;

they used to be on my husband's and my case when they were younger: "Get that cigarette; I can't stand smoke." But when they started the drugs, I think automatically all people who do crack cocaine also smoke. They can put the crack cocaine in a cigarette; that is how a lot of people start off.

I think a lot of people thought that when my husband died I would be smoking again. I wanted to, but then something just told me, "No, don't smoke. It's not going to bring him back, not going to solve anything." I am so glad I didn't pick that cigarette up. It was hard; it took everything this last time to not go back to smoking.

We were married thirty-seven years before he was killed right on the corner. It was two days after Thanksgiving. He was retired 'cause his health was bad. He was alcoholic. He left the house early in the morning. He was expecting his bonus check from the union. Usually when he sees the mailman come, he'll come back and have me sign the checks, so I can go to the bank. That particular day when the mailman came past, he never came here, so I looked out and there he was still on the corner, and I was looking at him. He was outside by a car, talking to somebody. I went into the bathroom and then, all of a sudden, I heard these *pop, pop, pop, pop, pops*. I went back to the window and looked again and then I see these legs sticking out into the gutter. I said, "Oh no, that is Charles." I went and got in my bed and I balled up into a knot. Somebody came and rang my doorbell and said Charles had been shot. I didn't go down there because I didn't want to see him lying out there, and I didn't know if he was dead.

I got on the phone and called my older sister. She came and took me to the hospital; he died on the operating table. They said on the death certificate that he had been shot multiple times. We had been here twenty years. Ever since we moved here, I always told him to stay off that corner. I used to always tell him that he was going to die on that corner, but I was just talking, I didn't really think that would actually happen.

He would have loved to have known that he had a grandbaby. When I found it out, I was devastated 'cause I didn't want her to have no kids in that state. I am glad the baby is here now. She was a month early. She was saying, "I want out." She is under my legal guardianship. She is doing well. My daughter cannot legally have her anymore until she [has] a year program behind her, and she has to go to parenting classes. She was not ready to be a mother, which I really hated because I thought she should have had a bond with her baby. She did not have that bond.

When I had my children, that was beautiful, but having my granddaughter: that, to me, is amazing. It is just wonderful. I never thought that this could be like this. I feel good about having her in my care 'cause I know somebody is taking care of her. Now, I've got plenty of energy, and I need it most definitely with my grandbaby. She is thirteen months. And I need all the energy I can get 'cause she is a handful.

I don't know what took me so long to quit smoking. I smoked for over thirty some odd years. I feel better. My appetite is better; I enjoy my food much, much more. I can take my time and eat, not in a big rush, so it has really helped. The doctor could feel my esophagus, but he can't do it anymore. I had stomach problems; I used to take all kinds of medications. I don't take medications anymore. I know it is a change, and it is due to not smoking.

Most places you go now, you cannot smoke, and I am so happy for that. If you could, maybe I might've gone back to smoking. That is what happened to me once before. I was arguing with my husband; he laid his pack of cigarettes on the table, and I just took one out and went downstairs and lit it. It just went on and on. I used to make excuses to go to the store to get things, so I could walk around the block to smoke. I thought I was fooling them. I thought that they didn't know I started smoking, but I was only fooling myself. My daughter caught me one day smoking and then everybody knew.

Now she knows I am serious, and she tells everybody: "My mother used to rather smoke than eat. Rather smoke than do anything, but I know she is not smoking now."

It works with the drugs, too. They say you work with the program and you quit and you go out and you go back to drugs, and then you go back and eventually it will kick in. I don't want to give up on my daughter, and I think one of these days it is going to kick in for her. If I continue with not smoking I think it will give her a little more encouragement to get off those drugs.

I think a lot of people want to quit, but they don't have the nerve or the will to quit. It has been five years and every 23rd of the month is my anniversary for not smoking. If I took one puff, I knew I would go back to smoking; if I took a drag, I would be draggin' forever. I just count the days and the months that I am not smoking. I celebrate every day; I buy lottery tickets; I just feel happy that I don't smoke; I really do.

"I celebrate every day; I buy lottery tickets; I just feel happy that I don't smoke; I really do."

I don't know what would happen to make me go back to smoking, I truly don't. If my husband's death didn't do it, and my kids out there didn't do it, especially that girl. She is out there somewhere, and you don't know where she is or what she is doing. It is devastating to me. Sometimes I wake up in the night; I go to the window just wishing for her to come, so I can know where she is. But I try not to let it bother me too much 'cause I can't stop it. She is a grown woman making her own choice, just like I have to make mine. But I just hate it.

Things have been a little more calm; I have been accepting things instead of getting all hyper. I have been accepting things like they are and not worrying about it. I made up my mind, that "What is the point?" 'Cause I was working myself into an early grave, and I have to be here to raise this baby. I want to be here until she gets to be an older child. I am hoping I live long enough. I just hope I will. I know I don't want to be getting to the point where I can't breathe or I can't chase her around. I know that by me not smoking, that is one way.

What moved Mary to be a non-smoker?

Mary had real opportunities to rationalize her smoking; after all, in her home, she was surrounded by smokers who had no investment in supporting her to stop. But Mary wanted to be successful at quitting smoking to prove that making really tough changes is possible. In her process, she used and developed personal resources like self-discipline and determination that carried her through hardships that would break many of us.

Instructions for life: Pay attention. Be astonished.
Tell about it. **Mary Oliver**

Paul Brunetta

Paul Brunetta, M.D., co-author of this book, is a doctor anyone would be blessed to have as a physician. Brilliant, creative, and dedicated, he has an uncanny ability to discover another person's capacities and draw them out. He possesses that rare capacity for full attention, and when he focuses his attention in your direction, you feel heard, seen, and appreciated. In all the years we have been friends, I have known him to be someone who leans into developing plans and projects that can benefit the greatest number of people. This book would not exist were it not for his insistence that the handful of photocopied stories and photographs I shared with him were the beginnings of a book, not just a packet of simple handouts. It was his vision that saw the scope of this project and how to develop it into a form that would reach as many smokers as possible.

Paul is dedicated to saving lives. All the work he applies himself to as a physician is in service of that goal. While he is tremendously effective in person-to-person interactions, his attention simultaneously includes the invisible mass of people dealing with any particular medical issue. In the case of smokers, he is on the lookout for any way he can help to reach the most people possible with skills and information they can use to free themselves from tobacco dependence.

Paul holds himself to a high standard. His parents were hard-working and he inherited no special privileges or luxury. He learned from an early age to work hard, to value family, and to live with integrity and principles. Happening onto smoking at an early age as part of his relationship with his beloved grandfather, he had a mixed and romantic association with tobacco. His experimentation further developed in the context of a best-friends relationship that has lasted into adulthood. For some considerable span of time, he was in denial over the increasing hold that cigarettes had over him. Like many other smokers, he operated under the illusion that he was not addicted and that he would be able to quit at any time he chose. By the time he finally faced the incompatibility of smoking with being a doctor, he was undeniably dependent on tobacco. His determination to become smoke-free grew out of a realization that being a smoker was essentially, for him, an expression of dishonesty. If he was not in complete alignment with his values and ideals, he could not reflect integrity as a doctor and a human being. Moreover, being under the control of cigarettes was unacceptable.

Many people who follow the challenging road to becoming smoke-free discover elements to value in their history as smokers. Paul mined the years of his relationship with tobacco to enrich and deepen his practice, helping others to achieve the freedom he found. As a doctor, he is in an especially powerful position to support people wanting to effect change. Many times, I witnessed an automatic rise in the self-esteem of smokers when they discovered that the M.D. leading their Group had also been tobacco dependent. If Paul had been hooked on tobacco, it must mean this really was a chronic disease and not a character flaw or weakness.

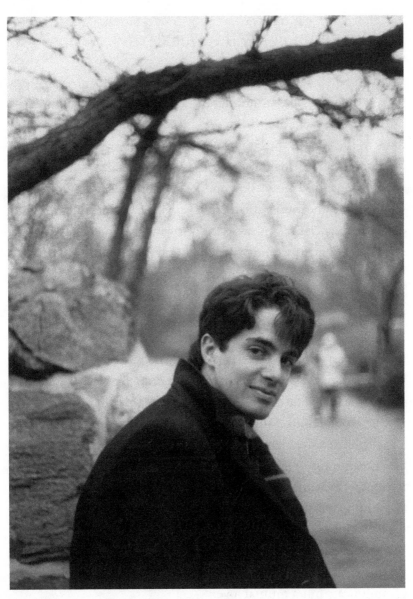

Paul Brunetta stopped smoking in his twenties.   Photo by courtesy of the author

Paul Brunetta, in His Own Voice

I grew up in a small town about fifty miles north of New York City and come from an immigrant-minded family. My mother is one of thirteen children from a very poor family in London and came to the U.S. in the late 1950s. My father is an only child from immigrant Sicilian parents with the same mentality—hard work, achievement, and education are top priorities in an uncertain world. My father went off to college, got a business degree, and did well financially; and as I was growing up in the sixties and seventies, I remember, he occasionally smoked a pipe or cigar. My Italian grandfather would smoke really cheap White Owl cigars. He had hypertension and later multiple small strokes; he was told to stop smoking in the last decade of his life.

When I was six or seven years old, my grandparents moved into an apartment over the garage right next to our house. Years later, when I was a young teenager, my grandfather would ask me to come over and bring a cigar, and when I did, we used to sit together and he would smoke and talk to me in broken English. We had an unspoken agreement that if I'd bring him an occasional cigar, he'd give me a little glass of peach brandy. He'd be so delighted—I remember the smile on his face, the click of his old Zippo lighter as he'd unwrap that cigar and light up. When I smell cigars now, there's an instant memory of Papa—that's what we used to call him. There's something very comforting about it and a unique memory I share with him—just sitting together with a limited ability to communicate but a mutual love.

Tobacco and smoking were familiar to me during that time. The Surgeon General's report was issued in 1964, and during my childhood, there were cigarette ads in all of the magazines—there were ads on TV. I was exposed to tobacco relatively early, but there was also a sense from my family that this was not healthy, and you shouldn't be smoking cigarettes. Pipes, cigars rarely might be okay, but cigarettes were definitely to be avoided.

I had my first cigarette when I was nine years old, and I remember it so vividly. I was at Catholic communion classes with my friend Brian, at his house. Brian's mom was our teacher, and midway through the lesson, she'd take a cigarette break. It was a very intentional thing—removing herself from us and going outside for a smoke. We'd watch her through the kitchen window out on the back deck—she was clearly doing something only grown-ups were allowed to do. When she would come back in, she'd be a different person—really relaxed, affectionate, and just so happy that we were there. She had a pack of cigarettes in her purse, and I stole one of them—perhaps that was before we got to the eighth commandment.

I remember bringing the cigarette back home and smoking it out on our back deck and the incredibly powerful rush, followed by the realization: "That's why people smoke!" There wasn't anybody in our house who smoked, so Brian was my connection to the source, mainly at parties and camping trips. I lived in a small town, and we had a forest behind our house, so camping for us was getting gear together and then hiking for twenty minutes and finding a clearing in the woods. Brian started experimenting more when we were fifteen; and then from sixteen to eighteen, he was a regular smoker, increasing to about half a pack a day by his late teens. I wouldn't smoke during the week, but on the weekends and at parties, I'd bum them. If I was around somebody who had them, it would be two or three at once, just to get that strong buzz.

I don't think I got to the point as a teenager where my body was conditioned to the nicotine; it was still an intense rush. I was very conscious of the smell of tobacco on people's clothes and breath and hair, and I knew my parents would be suspicious, so I was very careful about the way I gained access to it. Once in a while wouldn't have been a big deal, but if I was smoking regularly, that would have been a serious problem at home. "Once in a while," for me, became almost every weekend. All the way through my last two years of high school, I felt I could take it or leave it, but if I had access to it and there weren't judges around, I would definitely be up for it. If the opportunity arose, I'd be excited to smoke, but of course I didn't think of myself as a smoker. High school was a stressful time, and there were ways in which hanging out and sharing a cigarette was really enjoyable. I had ambitions and knew what I wanted to do, and I was very competitive. It was a nice escape, a stress reliever, and sort of a numbing agent. It was also part of an intense bonding experience. If you're with somebody who's a smoker and you're in an environment where smoking is not accepted, you feel like you're committing a minor crime together.

> "There was work and there was reward, and cigarettes became part of my reward system on a daily basis."

Going to college was the first time I had complete independence. I was kind of shy, but smoking and drinking are social lubricants. I was working really hard, studying for exams, and pulling all-nighters from intense premedical courses. It seemed to help me with anxiety and focus. Freshman to sophomore year, I converted from smoking on the weekends to a couple a day, and I was actually buying my own packs—in my mind, that was a completely new relationship to cigarettes. I was using them more frequently, getting acclimated to them, but I tried to limit my use to a couple a day. "That's not very much compared to people who smoke a pack a day," I'd tell myself.

Smoking was intensely enjoyable, and it helped me concentrate, so it had a place, but I thought I could control it. There was work and there was reward, and cigarettes became part of my reward system on a daily basis. I saw it more as a positive than a negative. There were regular cycles where exams were coming up, stress was building, and it wasn't just a couple a day. I remember coughing a lot, but I was firmly convinced I could max out at ten to fifteen a day, and that after exams were over, it would be a few a day. And then I got to the point where I had a couple of quit attempts that were associated with withdrawal symptoms. My anxiety level would go up—I'd get easily angry or morose, and I'd convince myself that having a cigarette was fine "for now." So, why? Why bring it down to a couple a day? What's the motivation? Why does it have to be fewer than fifteen? Why does it have to be zero? I reasoned that if I was able to go from ten to two, or even able to handle a couple of days without any, it provided a false assurance that I wasn't addicted. "I'm smoking because I like them and I want them, and, of course, I can stop whenever I want." Cigarettes were becoming less of a reward and more a way to treat anxiety.

That went on for at least a couple of years. I felt as though I was using [tobacco] as a tool to help me navigate a tough situation—difficult premedical studies and a future in medicine that required exceptional academic performance and serious, committed focus. There were still a lot of positives surrounding it—having drinks with friends, after sex—it was intense. There are ways in which meals are good, but a cigarette after a meal for a smoker is fantastic. I was very capable of functioning, and "I could quit whenever I wanted—not a problem." But I had a persistent daily sense that smoking was not what I wanted to do.

I remember buying a pack of Marlboro lights after I swore to myself that I was going to quit. It felt like I was physically pulled into a corner store by my split and addicted personality—almost like an out-of-body experience. I knew that I shouldn't, but I had to get a pack. I remember going in and laying my money down and having my heart pound with the feeling, "I'm not supposed to be doing this but I'm doing it anyway." I remember getting disgusted by that, crunching up the pack, and throwing it in the garbage—and then going through the garbage to try to find a cigarette in the pack that wasn't destroyed enough so I could still smoke it.

I was objective enough to recognize, "Okay, I'm on my knees now and my hands are in garbage, and I'm finding this crappy old cigarette—this is not good." It took me a few years to quit, going through that cycle over and over again where I was smoking two, five, ten, and then I would have a quit attempt. It would take me a while to really drop down. I would drop down: two or five or none. Almost nothing during the week, and all of my smoking on the weekend. Going to parties and drinking alcohol would demolish any resolve I'd built up in my mind. For weeks, I'd be successful at quitting, and then some stressful issue would come up and I'd break down again and buy a pack. Or maybe I'd have a successful two weeks, and then that split personality would yank me to the corner store and I'd go get another pack. It was a real struggle. I remember writing letters to my friend Brian because we were both trying to quit, and we promised ourselves that we would.

I must have tried to quit ten, fifteen, twenty times. I developed a new method, which was if I bought a pack and smoked a cigarette, I'd put them under the faucet, get them wet, and then I'd smash them up and throw them in the garbage. Then I'd have to go and buy another pack, so I was buying a whole pack to smoke one cigarette. Part of my effective method of quitting was to change the lie I was telling myself. Before, my lie had been, "I am going to smash up these cigarettes and throw them away so I'm not going to smoke anymore." But in the back of my head, I knew I could go find one that wasn't fully broken—I would intentionally not smash them completely. I was able to recognize that this was a lie and I tried to find a different method. It was getting me to a final destination by my going off the road a lot but also making slow, minor modifications and progress— learning to quit. By now, I knew that I was addicted. And I knew I wanted to stop and occasionally had the strength to stop.

My thought process wasn't, "I want to stop now so I don't get lung cancer or heart disease." It was: "This is a bad, addictive substance," and I began to think about what tobacco companies really do. I was giving money to a company that sells products that cause disease—the exact opposite of the "First do no harm" credo of medicine. I began to actively look for information about smoking, and that provided some motivation. I was buying into something that ultimately wasn't good for anybody. That was part of the motivation; the other piece was the dishonesty around smoking: when you do something you know you're not supposed to do, and you tell yourself, "I'm just going to have one." I was never a committed smoker—more of a reluctant participant caught up in something that was difficult for me to control. There are a lot of ways in which social smokers consider themselves to not be real smokers—you're not a real smoker unless you buy cigarettes. You're not really a smoker until you put your money down. It was something I would reward myself with. Then there were times where my stress level elevated and I really needed it to help me cope, and then I'd become really disgusted with myself for having lost control. So, for a pack-a-day smoker, maybe the thought process is, "Wow, two packs a day is horrible, but a pack a day—you know, that's not so bad." It's all somewhat relative, and you lose control of the concept that it's a reward—it becomes a necessity instead.

What really motivated me was the desire to control my behavior. I was very goal oriented and wanted to see my goal through and be honest with myself. My self-esteem would drop after smoking, because I was doing something that was wrong and harmful. There seemed to be this point where the longer I was out from my last cigarette, the less intense the urges were. I was able to hold them up and say, "OK, *that's* an urge. That's what that is—it's not some split personality taking me into a store," and then trying to deal with it in a more mature way. I used exercise and deep breathing, and there

> "I became better at recognizing when I was getting stressed and treating it with a cigarette."

comes a point where you're slightly more wise than you were in your twenties. I became better at recognizing when I was getting stressed and treating it with a cigarette. I began recognizing that there were other ways to handle my stress and insecurity: exercise, trying to be more verbal in a relationship, or intentionally talking things through rather than escaping to smoke a cigarette. And then, for sure, medical school—I'd finally arrived where I was hoping I would go, and some of the tension about whether I'd make it in life began to dissipate. It was clear—medical school was *not* a good environment for smoking. The idea of being a smoking doctor was really unacceptable to me.

What moved Paul to be a non-smoker?

Having authority over his own destiny is important to Paul. He has always worked hard to achieve his goals and to be the best person and physician possible. As a respected and expert physician and researcher, he could not reconcile his personal and professional values with being a smoker. He used his capacity for discipline to move himself to success, always guided by a determination to develop and maintain healthy self-control.

What moves you to be a non-smoker?

Action steps for people who want to be smoke-free

The two things I probably hated the most about being hooked on cigarettes were that I was always afraid about what smoking was doing to me as well as what I would have to endure when I finally put my attention to quitting; and, as a smoker, I had low self-esteem as a mother and as a nurse. Being a smoker did not line up with what I believed would make me the best mother I could be, and I saw myself as a negative role model for my patients, coming to their bedside reeking of cigarettes. Bottom line, I was very scared about what I was doing to myself by smoking. I turned "I don't want to be afraid and guilty" into a positive statement of what I did want: "I want to be fearless and proud."

With as much detail as I could, I imagined what it would feel like to be fearless and proud. How would I hold my body to experience those feelings? What would I think about myself, what thoughts would I cultivate in my mind? Starting twenty-one days before my quit date, at every possible opportunity I imagined myself embodying both feelings, and I made little signs to put up around my house and in my car that read: "I am smoke-free, fearless, and proud." By continuously repeating this mantra, I reprogrammed myself to be in alignment with what I wanted to be true. These words became a powerful beacon of support that guided and sustained me through difficult withdrawals and challenging situations as I rebuilt my life as a nonsmoker.

One of the most effective steps you can take is to begin keeping a list of your

> "I made little signs to put up around my house and in my car that read: "I am smoke-free, fearless, and proud."

"want to" motivations. Sometimes it is easier to determine what you want by going through your awareness of what you do not want. Think about and write down why you *want to* stop smoking rather than why you *have to* stop.

Stopping smoking is hard enough without getting into a battle with yourself; it is important to be on your own team. Encourage yourself with positive reinforcement rather than berating yourself for being less than what you think you should be. Take a moment here and try out an interesting exercise. On the last page of this chapter, you'll see a way to start a list of as many things as you can that you don't like about being a smoker. Then think about what you will get by not smoking. For example, if you are tired of the hassle of maintaining a tobacco habit, imagine the sense of freedom and simplicity that comes when you quit. Keep adding to your list over the next days and weeks, building a case for embracing the new life you are choosing to create for yourself.

Another revealing experiment is to close your eyes and allow your mind to quiet as you follow the movement of your breath coming in and out of your body. Now, in your mind or aloud, say, "I *have* to stop smoking, I *have* to stop smoking." Repeat this phrase a few times, and as you do so, notice any body sensations and any thoughts or feelings that arise. What do you feel as you repeat, "I *have* to stop smoking"? Take a minute or two and jot down a few words to describe your experience with this exercise.

> On the last page of this chapter, write a list of as many things as you can that you don't like about being a smoker. Then think about what you will get by not smoking.

Now, closing your eyes again, say: "I *want* to stop smoking." Even though you might be ambivalent about stopping smoking, just pretend for a few minutes that you want to stop. Again, say the phrase a few times while bringing your awareness to any body sensations, thoughts, and feelings. What do you notice? Record a few words to describe your experience.

Saying: "I have to" could trigger feelings of tightness or restriction; you might even have feelings of panic or resistance or a sense of hopelessness. The mind can react with various forms of "*no*, I don't." On the other hand, repeating "I want to" can result in feelings of openness, of options. There is greater relaxation and a feeling of "Nobody is making me do this; it's *my* choice and I can do it."

Three Key Points

1. More than fear or negativity, clear and positive motivations for change can effectively move us toward freedom from smoking.

2. Motivations we choose for change become a foundation for growing strengths and skills.

3. The more personal a motivation is and the more passionately we feel about it, the more potent a force for change it can be.

NOTES

_____

_____

_____

_____

_____

_____

_____

_____

_____

_____

_____

_____

_____

_____

_____

_____

_____

_____

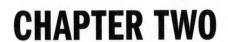

CHAPTER TWO

What do you like about smoking?

S topping smoking is a process, not an event. Early in the journey of becoming a non-smoker, you may find it helpful to explore your relationship with cigarettes in more detail. Having an understanding of what you like about smoking will support you in building an effective quit plan to let it go.

Many of us describe cigarettes as our best friend, always there when we need them. When we first fell into a relationship with this friend, it may have been exciting and allowed us to feel sexy, grown up, rebellious, or connected to a peer group. Then, as we matured, the relationship aged and became more complex. We discovered qualities we didn't like, leading us to consider breaking from the relationship. Smokers are often so used to the relaxing effect of a cigarette that they don't realize that the relaxation is just relief from nicotine withdrawal symptoms. The experience of reward and satisfaction is a remedy for the problem created by the cigarette itself.

You may have to fight a battle more than once to win it. **Margaret Thatcher**

Ernie Ring

Ernie Ring is a brilliant, powerful, world-renowned physician and radiologist, and perhaps more than any other person in this book, he is deeply familiar with the ravaging effects of tobacco use. Yet for years, smoking was a huge part of Ernie's persona. Even today, he freely admits that had there been no negative effects from smoking, he never would have stopped. But the x-rays he looks at every day are a constant reminder of what smoking does to the body.

Ernie was very clear about what he liked about smoking and the benefits he felt he had experienced from cigarettes. The ability to drive himself for long hours, to stay alert, and to have the mental sharpness to make life-and-death decisions for his patients were powerful reinforcers. In fact, he questions whether he would have been able to invent the radiological devices for which he is famous without the effects of nicotine. Further, he believes he would not have been able to work the long, grueling hours in interventional radiology without the stimulating effects of lots of cigarettes.

So, for Ernie, smoking was deeply intertwined with his sense of accomplishment, his work ethic, and his personality. People who knew Ernie knew him as someone who smoked; the two seemed inseparable. But there came a time when the price he was paying for smoking outweighed even the powerful benefits he enjoyed, and he was faced with the challenge of how to let go of such a fundamental part of who he was.

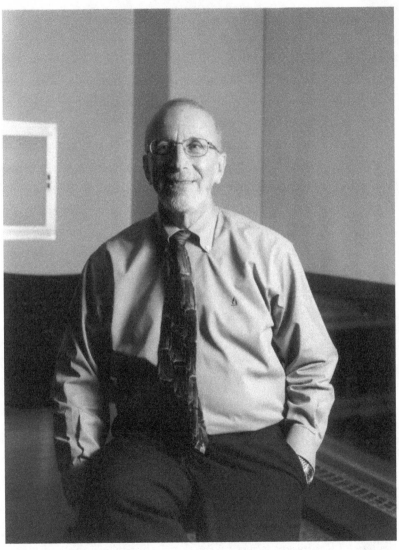

Ernie Ring   Photo by John Harding

Ernie Ring, in His Own Voice

I am currently chief medical officer for UCSF. It is a key position and an opportunity to play a role in how hospitals work and potentially to have a role in improving the overall care provided at UCSF to the thousands of patients we serve each year.

I graduated from medical school in 1969 and have been a practicing physician for 37 years. I received training in radiology at the Massachusetts General Hospital in Boston. I stayed on an extra year, as chief resident and a fellow in what was then called angiography, to get special training in the catheterization procedures that were done in the 1970s. I joined the faculty at the University of Pennsylvania in 1976 to head up the angiography section. As part of that experience I was put in a position to help innovate what became a new field of medicine, interventional radiology. We had a remarkable relationship with the surgery department, who saw the kinds of procedures that we were able to do under fluoroscopic guidance with catheters as an opportunity to be very innovative in practicing surgery. We worked together closely to expand this methodology into a major new approach to the treatment of surgical patients.

I eventually became president of a society that promotes interventional radiology. The creation of the society's journal took place in my office; the establishment of a foundation to support the research side took place over conference calls in my office. Then I became a member of the board of chancellors of the American College of Radiology, where I helped move interventional radiology from a group of procedures done by fearless and creative people to a field that is now practiced throughout the world. It has given me an opportunity to lecture on new procedures around the globe and to see them developed and become part of treatment in nearly every country on earth.

In 1997, I had my first heart attack. At the time, I was working eighty to one hundred hours a week at a job with enormous responsibility. I was not only engaged in complex procedures but also expected not to have failures or complications, and that meant I had to oversee every procedure done by my colleagues. It was a very gratifying time, a very difficult time, and, eventually, it overwhelmed me physically.

I started smoking when I was fifteen, primarily because that's what everybody did. It was in the 1950s, and smoking was the norm. I quickly became addicted. There was nothing wrong with it. It was accepted. Throughout the 1960s and 1970s, smoking in the hospital was standard practice. In those days, there was no digital imaging, so to see what you were doing with these procedures, you took frequent breaks to interpret films and evaluate your progress. Everyone would light up outside the processor while waiting for the film. I would smoke two packs on those eighteen-hour days.

"I was concerned that smoking was something I could rely on as a benefit when I needed it: clarity of thought for re-energizing at two or three in the morning."

In the 1980s, as society gained a better understanding of the dangers of smoking, more and more restrictions on smoking were imposed and social unacceptability grew. Between 1980 and 1990, smoking went from being pretty normal and socially acceptable to being something that could not be done around others, and totally unacceptable. By 1990, I was smoking surreptitiously in my office.

When I had the heart attack in 1997, it was a reaffirmation of what I already knew. The primary disease that I treat is peripheral vascular disease, but everybody I treat is a smoker. I would tell my patients that I smoke, and I would tell them that they had the disease and I didn't. Then I would tell them to quit smoking because the disease was only going to get worse; the people who had never smoked who told them to quit didn't understand what I was asking them to do. But I did understand. I recognized how hard it was to quit, and when I finally got the disease, I would have to quit too.

I really enjoyed smoking. I truly believed that it helped me to think. It was widely known among the people who trained with me that when a case was difficult or going badly, I would go into my office and come out with a solution to the problem. I was concerned that smoking was something I could rely on as a benefit when I needed it: clarity of thought for re-energizing at two or three in the morning. I saw it as a great benefit—a great risk, yes, but also a great benefit. I enjoyed it to the extent that it became relatively easy to deny the risk to continue to achieve the benefit. I continued to feel that way after my first heart attack right up until my second one in 2003. At that point, I decided to quit. But it was extremely difficult: the physical addiction, the mental dependence, the overall feeling of clarity I believed it gave me when I needed it, the absence of friends to turn to. I was the expert, and smoking was both a crutch and a friend that were very real to me. Giving that up in the complicated world in which I lived was tough. The mechanism ultimately involved lots of nicotine.

The mornings were the hardest, and moments of decisiveness were difficult.

I liked everything about smoking. In the early years, I liked the camaraderie associated with it. I liked the time-out nature of it. I liked the taste of it. It was part of my persona. Take me or leave me. I am really good at being who I am. I am really good at what I do. It is my business, not yours. After my second heart attack, my wife insisted that I quit smoking, and her reasoning was solid: only a fool would continue to smoke after two cardiac events. Up to that point, it had been almost part of a caricature of me: most people knew me as a smoker and recognized me from afar even if all they could see clearly was a cigarette. But once the second heart attack demonstrated the damage smoking was causing me, it would have only been a demonstration of some pretty dumb behavior to continue. That fact was highly motivating.

I finally got somebody at Stanford to say, "Just keep putting patches on until you feel comfortable," which took the process from impossible to just very difficult. That lasted probably nine months. I augmented the patches with nicotine gum as needed, despite wearing three patches at once at one point. Eventually, I got off the patches. I was in no rush. It took more than two years before I didn't think about smoking all the time.

Once I made the decision to quit, I saw it as an enormous challenge. I was willing to give up everything that I had been for the past 40 years to become whatever I would be as a smoke-free person. The challenge was more than just giving up a profound addiction. It was also the willingness to accept everything that came with that.

Everything discourages smoking now. There is no reason to start. In most of society, it is totally unacceptable. Of course, there may be some sense of leadership or uniqueness associated with smoking, just as there is with tongue piercing or tattooing, all practices that fit into a similar "outside-the-norm" category. But that's not the way it was 45 years ago, and I think that is an important change.

The key message now is to stay away from smoking in the first place. There is no reason to start, and it is so hard to undo once it is done. The cost, the stigma, and the labeling associated with smoking will have devastating implications for your entire life. I didn't have that when I started. It was okay to have the ambition I had to be an important, leading physician and to be a smoker. That is no longer true. If you choose to smoke today, your future will be subject to constraints. It is not the health side that is going to keep you from smoking; you have to wait too many years to feel the effects of that. The thing that makes you feel badly is the stigma. When you think highly of yourself and success is measured in a lot of different ways, smoking in an overachieving world is a symbol of underachievement.

What did Ernie Ring like about smoking?

Ernie was clearly aware of the drug effects of nicotine, and these were what he liked about smoking. If another drug was substituted in his story, such as cocaine, the effects he valued could be similarly experienced. It's impossible to imagine that he would defend using cocaine, however, or that he would willingly connect his professional successes to its use. Of course, there is no way to test his assumption that he would have been less successful as a non-smoker. When it came down to a decision, he knew that there was something he valued more than anything he got from smoking: his identity and reputation as an intelligent physician. Facing a very real threat to his health and life, along with consideration for his wife, he finally made the decision to take on the challenge and become smoke-free.

It's not the load that breaks you down, it's the way you carry it. **Lena Horne**

Roger Sako

Roger was born in a Japanese internment camp in the early 1940s. His father had worked at a dry cleaner, and his mother was a keypunch operator. It was common for Japanese men to smoke, and Roger enjoyed bonding with his dad through smoking. Over the years, Roger's life became more solitary; uncomfortable in most social situations, he found comfort and a sense of companionship with cigarettes.

Roger was notable for his quiet presence and striking appearance: he had long, thick black hair reaching to his waist. His doctor referred him to our program because daily smoking was worsening his other chronic health problems. Roger had been cutting down on cigarettes by rolling his own. When he explored what he actually liked about smoking, he discovered that he didn't enjoy that many of the 30 cigarettes he smoked each day. The biggest pleasure was found in the first cigarette of the day and the one he smoked after each meal. Any other pleasure came from satisfying the nicotine urge or relieving boredom.

I had known Roger for less than two years. In our first meeting, he timidly said that he would not participate in any Groups. Painfully shy, he couldn't tolerate being in a room with more than one or two people. At the same time, he was determined to stop smoking and felt he couldn't do it on his own, so we arranged to meet one on one.

Roger lived in a residential hotel. His health problems drastically limited his energy, so he spent a lot of time alone in his room. He felt so lousy that it took a huge effort to keep appointments, but he came faithfully to every one, always having practiced the suggested skills. Due to his committed effort, he became smoke-free within a few weeks. He was determined not to relapse, so we agreed to keep meeting on a regular basis until he felt confident that he could remain a non-smoker.

One afternoon, Roger showed up for our scheduled visit clearly very anxious. Shaking and stuttering, he told me that his doctor had just informed him that he had lung cancer. I was shocked by this news, but what happened next surprised me nearly as much: Roger wanted to come with me that night to Group so that he could be an example to the people who were still smoking. He wanted to convince people to stop smoking before it was too late, before they had to face what he was facing.

Over the next weeks, Roger started treatment for lung cancer. His beautiful long hair fell out in clumps until only a few wisps remained. He began losing weight at an alarming rate, shrinking from 181 pounds to 139 pounds in less than three months. Tumors in his brain gave him pain so severe that even heavy doses of narcotics did not give him relief. Terrified and lonely, Roger wasted away before my eyes—and yet a new strength emerged.

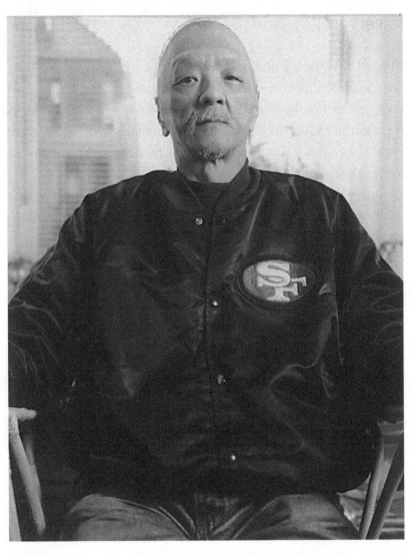

Roger Sako

Photo by John Harding

Roger Sako, in His Own Voice

When I first started smoking, there were no warnings about lung cancer, about nicotine being the most addictive substance on earth, about how you can get gum disease and die from smoking. Back in the 1950s, they [the tobacco companies] used to advertise everywhere—on TV, billboards, radio—but they never mentioned anything about how smoking could kill you.

My dad smoked like a chimney. I remember him going to a vending machine, sticking in a quarter, and when the pack came out, two or three pennies would be inside the cellophane wrapper—your change was already in the pack. What he'd do is give the pennies to me and my two sisters. Back then—that was the late 1940s and early 1950s—a couple of pennies and you were rich. I was so young that I didn't think about smoking. I just wanted the money.

When I started smoking, I was fifteen or sixteen. Everybody, all the people I ran around with, we smoked. We used to play poker, and we didn't have that much money, so we would play for cigarettes.

If you want to quit smoking, you have to be disciplined; you have to really commit yourself. Right off, when you wake up, you want that cigarette. And you think it is pleasure that you get from smoking it. That pleasure is both kind of real and kind of an illusion: It's real because you know you're satisfied, but it's an illusion because all you're doing is satisfying your nicotine urge, to get that nicotine level back up in your blood.

No matter how much pleasure smoking gives you, it's not worth it. You have to wrestle with that in your mind, because smoking is so addictive. I always thought, "My dad smoked all his life, he never got cancer, so I'm not going to get it," and then boom: I started losing weight, I had pain in my chest, and I couldn't swallow, so I went down and got a chest x-ray. That's when the lung tumor showed up. It came right out of the blue. I never expected it. Boom—it hit me just like that, with no warning. I was in the hospital for eight days; the last day I was there, I had my first chemotherapy, and then I started my radiation therapy. I got brain tumors because the lung cancer spread. They shrank, but the doctor tells me they can always come back.

I try not to think about dying, but it's difficult because I'm run down, I'm tired all the time, it hurts to breathe or swallow, and I have trouble maintaining my weight. I have to take pills to get an appetite. It's hard to make yourself eat when you don't feel like eating. It's probably one of the hardest things to do.

"I think half of the reason that people don't believe that smoking is bad is because you're fine for a long time."

Every day, I'm just surviving. I take my medication and hope it's doing some good. It's been almost six months since I was diagnosed. Doctors have told me six to eight months, max. In August, I asked, "Will I see another Super Bowl?" I want to see the 49ers win one more Super Bowl. But that six-to eight-month period, it's coming pretty quick now.

I think half of the reason that people don't believe that smoking is bad is because you're fine for a long time. It took 35 years for me to develop that cancer. Some 100,000 men and women get lung cancer every year. It all has to be from smoking. I went back to the [smoking-cessation] Group to see if I could get through to people because they could end up like me. Three people who heard me tell my story quit smoking.

If you're smoking, get your head straight and quit. It's just not worth it to go through the pain and the misery that I'm going through. Once you have cancer, your whole life is completely turned around. It's geared only toward survival for the time you have left, and nothing is normal anymore. The pleasure you get from smoking versus what I have … there's just no comparison. It's just not worth it. It's gonna cost me my life.

What did Roger Sako like about smoking?

Like many smokers, Roger had never examined his assumption that he smoked because he enjoyed it. When he directly questioned that assumption, he discovered that any cigarettes that were actually enjoyable were certainly not worth the price he ultimately played for that pleasure: his life.

There is no large and difficult task that cannot be divided into little easy tasks. **Buddhist Saying**

Sonya Hotchkiss

Sonya grew up on a turkey farm. By her own report, she had a wholesome and happy country childhood. She remembers that when she was a young girl, smoking made her feel glamorous. Years later, when she came to Group, she was smoking two to three packs a day and no longer feeling glamorous. Even so, she insisted she still liked smoking. With encouragement, she decided to look at what had started her smoking and what she enjoyed about it now.

Even though Sonya was smoking 40 to 60 cigarettes a day, she discovered she really only enjoyed smoking about six of them: the first two at the start of the day, the ones after each of her meals, and the last one at night. She realized that she was mostly smoking to keep herself out of withdrawal, not because she enjoyed it. When faced with the reality that she didn't actually like smoking most of the cigarettes she smoked every day, and because she was experiencing significant health problems associated with smoking, she said, "If I knew then what I know now, I would have been crazy to start smoking." Once she finally did stop smoking, Sonya was like many smokers in the program: when they really look at what they're doing and how they feel about it, the reality is starkly different from the story they have been telling themselves over the years.

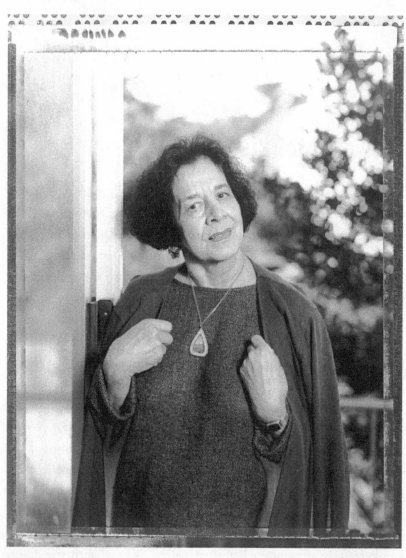

Sonya Hotchkiss

Photo by John Harding

Sonya Hotchkiss, in Her Own Voice

I was born in Brockton, Massachusetts, in 1935. I am the middle child of five kids. We lived on the outskirts of town on a turkey farm. My father was employed in a local shoe factory and my mother worked the farm.

I was kind of rebellious. I belonged to the Methodist Youth Fellowship (MYF). We went to the leader's house one weekend, and a friend of mine who was there taught me how to smoke. It was so important for me to learn. It was the thing to do. I had to do it right. I wanted to look more grown up, to be glamorous like Bette Davis. I was fifteen, in the tenth grade. We were up in the bedroom, doing it near a window. I learned on Lucky Strikes. Just before dinner, I inhaled for the first time. I got really dizzy, I was nauseated, and it was dinnertime. Then, of course, it got easier.

I don't think my mother knew that I smoked in the house. I remember smoking in my room and having a wet towel to fling around in the air. I thought that would take away the smoke. Smoking really stinks. My room smelled all the time. When I was in the house, it would be okay, but if I went out and came in, it would hit me.

Twenty years ago, I went in for a yearly physical and the doctor told me he couldn't believe how much I smoked and how beautiful my lungs were. That was the worst thing he could have told me; not too long after that, I had a chest x-ray and it showed that I was pre-emphysemic. I kept on smoking because I didn't seem to have any symptoms; it was just something in a picture on an x-ray. I smoked at least two packs a day, if not three. There was always a lit cigarette somewhere near me. As soon as one went out, I lit up the next one.

For the last two years before I stopped smoking, I was getting colds, and they would end up in my ear. Then I would turn deaf because the cold would plug up my Eustachian tube. The ear, nose, and throat doctor said that if I stopped smoking, that problem would possibly go away, which turned out to be true. When I stopped smoking, I didn't get a cold for two years.

The first time around, I kept in mind that I was just practicing stopping. Smoking is one of the more difficult things to give up. It is horrendous.

I cut down during our smoking-cessation Group. I wrapped up my cigarette pack in a piece of paper so that [whenever I smoked,] I had to unwrap the pack. Then I wrote down what I was doing and the stress level of it. In the morning, I put off unwrapping the pack for fifteen minutes. [Tapering] can be done, but I was really only stopping for fifteen minutes. I didn't want to do that all the time. How many times a day was I stopping? I couldn't light up when I wanted to, so what I was doing was like stopping and that was agony. Feelings arose. They weren't pushed down, so I was more aware of my feelings.

One of the things that helped was going back each week to the [smoking-cessation] Group and hearing stories of the difficulties others were having. The self-hypnosis tape worked too. I used it when I went to bed at night and took time to listen to it during the day. It helped me to not climb the walls, psychologically. It took a lot of anxiety away. Every time the craving came, I would count backward from eight to zero, and by the time I got to zero, the desire was totally gone. My mind was blocked; it could not think about cigarettes. [Counting backward] really did unplug everything in my head to do with cigarettes.

A month before my cutoff date, I switched from regular coffee to decaf because I didn't want to go through the withdrawal of coffee

"I think the thing that really helped was cutting back on cigarettes, then limiting myself to a certain number each day, and finally just quitting."

and cigarettes. When I stopped smoking, I switched to tea. Now I drink ginger tea. I have coffee when I go out. I think the thing that really helped was cutting back on cigarettes, then limiting myself to a certain number each day, and finally just quitting. Everything clicked at just the right time.

It is really great that I do not have to unplug myself and be interrupted to light a cigarette and then stink up the whole place and myself. It is a sense of freedom. I don't feel that my life is centered around my cigarettes, which it was before. I didn't realize until now how much cigarettes were my life.

I don't want to get complacent. That would be dangerous. It was a bad addiction. Looking back, I see that it was easy to take stopping a day at a time. For me, anticipating stopping smoking was worse than actually doing it. I didn't like smoking anyway.

I didn't realize that the smell of my addiction would go through my whole being. I am still Sonya, but now I am Sonya who doesn't smoke.

What did Sonya Hotchkiss like about smoking?

Like Roger, when Sonya examined her smoking experience, she discovered that she enjoyed only a few of the forty to sixty cigarettes she smoked every day. What had started out as something to make her feel sexier and attractive became something that left her smelling like stale smoke. Many smokers are unaware of how strongly the residue of their smoking smells. It's not until sometime after they've quit and have begun to regain their normal sense of smell that they detect the strong tobacco odor in their closets, on their clothing, and in their cars. As smokers, they had attempted to mask this odor with strong perfumes, colognes, and aftershave, unaware they were walking around enveloped in an unpleasing mix of stale tobacco and too much cover-up.

What do you like about smoking?

Action steps for people who want to be smoke-free

Ernie attributed his professional success to smoking, a reward that has deeper impact than glamour. He credits smoking with maximizing the power of his brilliant mind; he felt ready to quit when he understood that he did not want to see himself as stupid for continuing to smoke after two heart attacks. To tolerate major withdrawal symptoms and continue working, he elected to consult a physician/tobacco-treatment specialist who prescribed multiple nicotine patches and nicotine gum.

If you consider that every reason we have for smoking is a "good" one but that the smoking itself is a problem, you may find it worthwhile to **look at your personal reasons for smoking**. If you like smoking because it makes you feel glamorous or sexy, how else might you feel those things in a way that would not threaten your health? Can you imagine the fun you might have getting creatively involved in experiencing your glamour and sexiness? You might want to color your hair, purchase some stylish clothing, or take tango lessons. You might put yourself in a new social situation where no one knows you and you are free to reinvent yourself with a new, fun style.

If you like cigarettes because they help you to relax, what are some healthier stress-reducing options? Perhaps a yoga class, some herbal tea, or meditation? When we become aware of what we like about smoking, we are free to find something that could, ultimately, be more satisfying. For example, I was aware that I really enjoyed the ritual of pulling the pack out of my purse, tapping out a cigarette, and lighting up. A lot of hand gestures associated with smoking gave me pleasure. When I stopped smoking, I needed to find other means of expression to satisfy the needs that cigarettes had filled. Some things were very simple, like making a ritual of lighting a candle and preparing herbal tea, which I enjoyed quietly. Sometimes I would sit and light incense and watch the patterns made by the smoke as it rose in the air. Needing something substantial to take the place that smoking had held in my life, I explored creative pursuits like sculpting and ultimately began painting. When I look back at my life and weigh the pleasure I got from cigarettes and the satisfaction I get from painting, there is no contest. Painting demands an investment of myself; it is a direct expression of myself. Smoking just took my breath away.

Roger Sako was confronted with a decision none of us would welcome: to live smoke-free with lung cancer or to revert to smoking. The choice to stay smoke-free in such highly stressful situations requires commitment and discipline. Roger was clear that what he wanted from being a non-smoker was more important to him than the discomfort he felt from withdrawal. He wanted the experience of being in charge of something in his life, of reclaiming his power from the very behavior that threatened to take away his life.

There are many things to like about smoking: the ritual of taking out and lighting the cigarette, the enjoyment of watching the smoke slowly uncurl in the air, the ability to use a smoke as an excuse to take a break or leave an uncomfortable situation. We enjoy cigarettes after meals, when we're upset, when we're celebrating. What we enjoy is usually outweighed by what we lose, however, as Roger discovered after he decided to quit. Like many people who get a life-threatening diagnosis from smoking, Roger reevaluated the pleasure he had taken for granted and wished he'd not indulged in it for so many years.

On a scale of zero to ten, with zero being not at all important and ten being as important as it could be, how important is it for you to stop smoking?

Each of us takes a different path to arrive at a strong decision to stop smoking. On a scale of zero to ten, with zero being not at all important and ten being as important as it could be, how important is it for you to stop smoking? What could make it more important? It doesn't take a life-threatening diagnosis to bring yourself to the point of commitment. Take a moment to jot down a few thoughts about how you might build your determination to stop smoking. What are some ways you can help yourself commit to quitting?

Some people insist that if they got a diagnosis of lung cancer, they would start smoking again right away: why not? Roger made a different choice. There wasn't much he could do about dying, but he could do something about how he was going to live out the rest of his days. He chose to make meaning out of his predicament and to try to save others from his fate.

Roger became very clear about his denial story. It was, "It can't happen to me." Unfortunately, while we have some choice about whether or not to smoke, we have no choice about what smoking might do to us. Given this reality, when you look into your own future, what do you see? What choice do you want to make? Take a few minutes to jot down some thoughts about where you would like to be in six months or a year.

The gift of Roger's story is that he became passionate about helping other people avoid the suffering that he was experiencing. He wanted to help others make different choices than he made. Can you imagine feeling passionate about protecting people you love by encouraging them to stop smoking? If so, then try turning toward *yourself* now with that same, supportive energy. Start by acknowledging yourself for reading this book and think about what you experience as support. Sometimes we can feel nagged or badgered by friends and loved ones who want us to stop smoking. The ways they approach us and talk about our smoking actually makes us want to escape and have a cigarette. What would support look like to you? Would it be positive messages giving you credit for your efforts? Would it be having your family not ask you about your quitting process? When I was stopping smoking, I paired up with a friend who was working on losing weight. We started out by telling each other precisely what kind of support we each wanted. I was clear that I wanted us to have a weekly check-in, and that if we saw each other between those times, she was not to ask me how I was doing. I wanted her to leave it up to me to bring up the subject if I wanted to. Then, during our check-in, I wanted her to help me remember the progress I was making, even if I was having setbacks.

"Many former smokers discover that having the opportunity to give back has helped them to stay smoke-free once they have stopped."

Because the "it can't happen to me" happened to Roger, he felt the urgent desire to wake up others to what he had been denying. You can receive people's best wishes and then move forward with caring for yourself in ways that will help you to stop smoking. Like me, you could choose to pair up with someone to share support. This could be someone who has already stopped smoking. Many former smokers discover that having the opportunity to give back has helped them to stay smoke-free once they have stopped. Your need for support to stop smoking could be a source of support to someone else who is working to stay smoke-free. If you are looking for other ways to build your determination to stop smoking, how about finding a Group or program where you can feel both supported and accountable? You could also talk to you doctor about medications that can help you through the early stages of quitting smoking.

Sonya Hotchkiss initially liked smoking because it helped her feel grown up and glamorous. In the stop-smoking program, she completed a simple exercise to better understand her relationship with cigarettes. She divided a blank piece of paper into four equal parts and then labeled the parts: good things about smoking, not-so-good things about smoking, not-so-good things about stopping smoking, and good things about stopping smoking. Doing this exercise, she discovered that over the years she had lost touch with early rewards and grew to feel more the burden of smoking. It actually felt more stinky than glamorous. Try the exercise now to explore what smoking does and doesn't do for you.

Good things about smoking	Not-so-good things about smoking
Not-so-good things about stopping smoking	Good things about stopping smoking

As much as Sonya had grown to dislike smoking, she found she could not just stop, so she decided to approach her quit date by tapering down on cigarettes. She wrapped the cigarette pack in a piece of paper, and each time she wanted a smoke she had to deal with the inconvenience of unwrapping the pack and writing down what she had been doing and what level of stress she was experiencing. You could try something similar. The simple step of making cigarettes a little more inconvenient often results in diminishing the number of cigarettes you smoke.

Three Key Points

1. The reasons why you first found cigarettes to be pleasurable and attractive may no longer be true for you after years of smoking.

2. After careful and honest investigation, many smokers discover that they actually enjoy only a small number of the total cigarettes they smoke.

3. When measured against the pain and suffering smokers experience from smoking, the pleasure they may have enjoyed becomes of questionable value.

NOTES

CHAPTER THREE

What is your denial story?

Denial can be helpful when it protects us from being overwhelmed by threatening information. Patients who are given very serious medical news will sometimes go into denial as a way to cope with too much fear and discomfort. This denial allows for taking in the information more slowly, allowing the person to manage very scary situations. But denial is harmful when it lets you keep doing something unhealthy like smoking. Some smokers put off dealing with uncomfortable feelings about their smoking for years and continue to smoke. In these cases, denial becomes whatever we tell ourselves to make it okay to keep on smoking.

Early in our stop-smoking program, we invite participants to explore their personal denial stories. Your story can be quite simple: "I can't stop." Or perhaps you have had a chest x-ray and your doctor pronounced that your lungs look clear, so you tell yourself that smoking is not causing you any harm. In fact, many of us hold the conscious or unconscious belief that smoking-related illness happens to someone else and not to us. Some smokers even tell themselves stories like "My sister got lung cancer and never smoked, so what is the difference? I may as well smoke." Another common denial story describes an elderly relative who smoked into his or her eighties or even nineties without consequence. The conclusion of these stories is always that it's okay to continue smoking.

Whatever your personal denial story, it's likely, when you try to quit smoking, that your mind will come up with some way of using that story to get you back to your old habit. Becoming aware of the story you've been telling yourself is the first step in eliminating its power to control you. If you're telling yourself that you just can't stop, perhaps it's because you've already made multiple attempts or you know that most people have to try several times before they are successful. You could, instead, tell yourself that you have yet to discover the treatment plan that is going to bring you to success and you will keep searching until you do. In the case of the clear chest x-ray, you could remind yourself that by the time a cancer shows up on an x-ray you are already in deep trouble, and instead of using a clear report as a reason to keep smoking, you could use it to say, "Wow, that's great, my lungs appear to be in good shape. I want to stop smoking and keep them that way."

In the example of a nonsmoking friend having lung cancer, a healthier supporting response might be: "That's an illness I want to do everything I can to avoid." Denial stories vary greatly and can be adapted over time. For example, you may know people who said in their twenties that they intended to quit smoking before their thirties, yet the timeline gets adjusted forward. Or a friend might say she is going to stop smoking when she finds a new job; the new job is secured, and then she tells herself that she's under too much stress to quit and she'll do it once she feels more at home in her work.

> Whatever your denial story, take a few minutes to write it down here. Bring it fully into your awareness. Doing so will rob it of its power and make your way to freedom clearer.

My Denial Story

_____

_____

_____

_____

_____

_____

_____

_____

_____

_____

_____

_____

_____

_____

_____

_____

_____

_____

_____

_____

_____

_____

Remember, you have two lives. You get your second life when you realize you have only one.
Pema Chödron

R.E.C.

R.E.C. had an effective denial story. Insisting she smoked "hardly at all," she was unconvinced of the importance of stopping completely. Except for a light smoking habit, her life was in balance and on track. She is active physically, socially, and politically. Swimming and walking help keep her fit; she also regularly enjoys cultural events and has worked several jobs. A highly intelligent woman with a friendly sense of humor, R.E.C.'s lively personality brought a sparkle to the smoking-cessation Group. Over a period of years, she attended intermittently. She was a great resource for low-cost and free activities to keep attendees busy and out of trouble.

After an absence of several months, R.E.C. again showed up to Group. Taking her turn to share, she announced with passionate conviction that she had had her last cigarette—ever. She went on to tell us that she had had a heart attack and was finally convinced that smoking in any amount was risky. Her denial story, "I'm not smoking enough for it to hurt me," had been shattered.

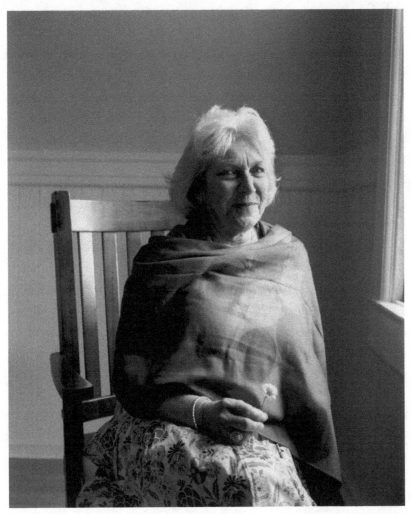

R.E.C.

Photo by John Harding

R.E.C., in Her Own Voice

Both of my grandfathers smoked. I have wonderful pictures from the 1930s of my grandfather in Amsterdam in a white linen jacket looking very bohemian, smoking. My father smoked; I loved the smell of smoking and I associated smoking with men who were strong and in control, whom I looked up to. When I was eleven or twelve, I would take my father's Camels or I would smoke butts. Then I found out other kids my age were smoking and they would come to my house after school and we would smoke. I smoked from then until I had a heart attack.

I wanted to quit smoking for many years. Most of my life, I smoked as many as ten cigarettes a day. I didn't get off of cigarettes by going to a cessation workshop. When the shit hit the fan, I would smoke a cigarette. I remember how that list of carcinogens and toxic elements in just one cigarette hit me, so I didn't want to do it. I cut down to even fewer each day. I had the heart attack at a time when I wasn't smoking very much.

In June 1999, I went to New York on a business trip and to see friends and family. I got there the day before Memorial Day. I got off the plane at Kennedy in a big, big heat wave. The Tuesday after the holiday, I was tired and it was very hot and I was drinking plenty of water, but I couldn't stop sweating from all my pores. I stayed at my friend's house all day. I didn't go anywhere. The next day, I went into the city, and then that night when I went to bed, I couldn't sleep. I had a cigarette in the middle of the night and that probably was the one I didn't need.

The next morning, Thursday, I had a noon appointment at the Oyster Bar at Grand Central Station. It was still really hot, even when I took a shower around 11 a.m. I got out of the shower and got dressed. I was sitting by the couch and suddenly I couldn't breathe, so I said to my friend, "I am going to lie down for a bit and see if I feel better." We had known each other since we were teenagers and she said, "You just don't look right. I'm calling 911." I told her not to call, but she called anyway and they came right away. I had TPA [a clot-busting medication used in heart-attack victims] in me within 40 minutes.

The Beth Israel Cardiac Unit and Angioplasty Lab is on 16th Street and I was on 91st Street, so I had to get transported. It took them from about noon until around 2:30 until they felt that I was stable enough to be moved. They told me, "You know you might die on the way downtown. We don't know. It is very dangerous to move you, but we have to." But I didn't die. That was Thursday. I had the angioplasty Friday morning at 9 o'clock.

Angioplasty was scary, and I was awake the whole time. There were all these people wearing masks, a big-screen television, and me on the operating table. My doctor was telling me what was going on: "Now we are going to cut open your groin, and now we are going to feed in a wire and the wire is going to have a balloon on the end of it." While I watched them messing around inside my heart with wires and things, I was thinking "Oh my God, how am I going to get through this? I can't take this."

My doctor was terrific. Finally, they were finished and he asked, "Now tell me. How did that feel?"

"Not very pleasant," I responded.

And then he asked, "How would you like to be here again?" I told him that I wouldn't think so, and he said, "I guarantee that if you continue to smoke cigarettes, you will be back here." That was it. That did it. It was a terrible experience, and although the procedure didn't hurt, it was creepy, and I didn't like it. I haven't smoked a cigarette since.

I had one occlusion in the artery of the lower right ventricle. I was lucky. They put a double stent in there. That was June 3 or 4, 1999.

"... he said, 'I guarantee that if you continue to smoke cigarettes, you will be back here.'"

My father, my brother, and both of my grandfathers had heart attacks. They have all died, and they were all smokers when they died. But I didn't think I was at risk because I didn't smoke that much and because I was so active. When I went to see the cardiologist afterward, he said, "What did you think, you were immune because you were a woman?" I never saw myself as a prime candidate for a heart attack. I thought I smoked so little and I had been a swimmer for many years, and so although I was a little heavier, I was still basically in pretty good shape. He told me that is why I lived, because the majority of women who have a heart attack at age 54 die right away. I feel fortunate that I did so well.

The whole experience was frightening. You don't have control over your body, and, for someone like me who likes being in control, that was upsetting. I had a hard time sleeping because I was under observation, and between not being able to sleep and the drips and other stuff stuck in my body, plus the possibility of having to go for an operation in the morning, I was terrified. My kids were 3,000 miles away, and I didn't know if I was going to live or not. I didn't know if I was going to go home to California or not. After the angioplasty, a big sand bag was laid on my groin over my femoral artery to ensure the incision did not open up. It remained there for six or eight hours and was not very comfortable. But then the next day I got out of the hospital.

I have recovered well, and I feel very lucky. That was a wake-up call for me, and everything was a gift from that point forward. I had symptoms of this heart attack before it happened. I couldn't breathe and I couldn't stand up straight. I had chest pain, but it didn't last long. When they first came and put me on the gurney, I said, "Gee, my left hand is tingly. Do you think I am having a heart attack? If I am going to be maimed for life because of this, just let me have a heart attack and let me die, because I don't want to be impaired."

One of them said to me, "Oh, you're strong as an ox and you're going to be just fine."

It is now a decade later. I didn't experience any damage thanks to a combination of quick attention, the TPA drug, and a wonderful cardiac hospital. I suspect that if the same thing had happened to me here in San Francisco, I would not be with you today because I would have gone back to bed. I would have ignored what I was feeling and not gone to the hospital. Heart attack symptoms can vary, especially for women. If you suddenly feel you are unable to breathe, do something about it. I was very fortunate.

What was R.E.C.'s denial story?

R.E.C.'s denial story is common among many smokers who smoke only a few cigarettes, or smoke infrequently. She carried the illusion that she was smoking too little for tobacco to actually hurt her. In fact, **there is no safe level of smoking**, just as there are no safe cigarettes. In playing Russian roulette, the blanks won't get us. Unfortunately, no one knows when the real bullet is going to fire.

Have patience. All things are difficult before they become easy. Saadi

Bill Andrews

Bill drove a San Francisco taxicab for 25 years. He smoked as a way to relax, to relieve boredom, and to control worry about whether he was going to make enough money. Coming into Group after work, he would immediately line up a series of inhalers that he used to relieve shortness of breath. Others in the Group urged him to set a quit date and prepare to stop smoking. But he came to Group irregularly, just often enough to fool himself into thinking that he was trying to quit but not so much that he would have to break through his denial about what he was actually doing. When his breathing worsened, Bill would simply increase his medications, feel better, and then go back to smoking up to three packs a day. He said he was aware of the risks he was taking but felt that having to go on oxygen was something that happened to other people, not to him.

It was painful and frustrating to witness Bill's decline as he continued smoking. When he eventually *was* put on oxygen, he had to cut back on cigarettes; he had to turn off the tank to smoke or run the risk of setting himself on fire. One day, he described a scary experience taking a road trip to Half Moon Bay, a town about forty minutes south of San Francisco. After lunch, he and his friend got back into their car to head home. They stopped at a traffic signal, and when the light changed; the car stalled. Bill's

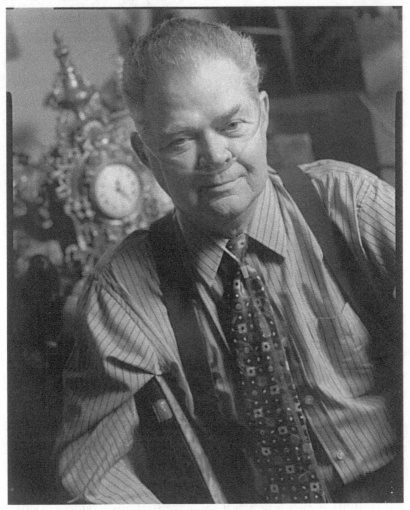

Bill Andrews

friend could not get the car started again. Bill had left home with four hours of oxygen in tanks and now had only one and a half hours left. When the tow truck arrived, the young driver couldn't handle the problem and had to call for help. By this time, Bill was down to thirty minutes of oxygen. With the car problem finally solved, Bill and his friend raced back to San Francisco, arriving home just as Bill ran out of oxygen.

It wasn't until Bill's cough got so bad that he couldn't smoke that he finally decided to quit. By then, he was on oxygen around the clock. Any activity had to be carefully planned and required help. If he wanted to go to the grocery store, someone had to go with him to help load and unload the groceries. He could no longer clean his home or do his own laundry, and he often ate his dinner out of a can because he didn't have the energy to cook.

When I interviewed Bill for this book, he had been smoke-free for two years. We met in his home, where everything was set up to minimize any effort to get his basic needs met. He was on a 20-foot hose attached to an oxygen concentrator so that he could get himself from the living room to the kitchen and bathroom. I could not suppress my tears when Bill described the joy he had felt as a young man running through the fields to school. Running, he said, was the only thing he'd ever felt good at. He had once dreamed of running the Bay to Breakers, a century-old San Francisco footrace. I felt heartache at the contrast between Bill's youthful freedoms as a runner and his current limitations based on how far he could move from his oxygen tank. Some of us get short of breath walking up hills and have to stop and rest; Bill couldn't even speak a full sentence without having to pause several times to catch his breath. Smoking had robbed him of the possibility of achieving his full potential.

Bill Andrews, in His Own Voice

I don't remember my first cigarette, but I know I snatched it from my dad because I wanted to be sophisticated. Being fourteen wasn't fun, and that summer my folks put me on a bus to stay with my grandparents. At the first bus stop, I got off and bought a pack of Camels. Grandma and Grandpa didn't like me smoking. They decided that if they let me have three cigarettes, maybe they could keep me from smoking too much. It didn't work.

I was a great cross-country runner. Hurdles, too. Where I grew up, there were a lot of open fields with stone fences. I would run through those fields and over those fences without even thinking about breathing hard. Going to school was a three-mile run. I would beat the school bus every time. I didn't know anything about the Olympics, or I might have tried out for it.

At that age, I wasn't really feeling any effects of smoking, but it wasn't long before it took its toll. Smoking slowed me down. I moved to San Francisco just as I was turning forty. On my fortieth birthday, I went to Stinson Beach [about 25 miles north of San Francisco] with some friends, and when we were running in the sand, I couldn't make it 20 feet. I was out of breath. I blamed it on the beer I was drinking and didn't try to run anymore. I decided to give up alcohol, but it didn't relieve the shortness of breath.

I began to realize that smoking was causing my breathing problems and I quit for a day or two. But there was no improvement, so I went back to smoking. After I was diagnosed with emphysema, I still didn't feel like quitting. I knew I should, but I really didn't want to quit. There were too many things going on in my mind, and smoking was a way of calming down, relaxing. The inhalers worked so well that I felt like I was cured. I had been smoking for a long time and I was not dead yet, plus it was easy to get treatment and feel wonderful. You start feeling so good and, knowing that your medications will help relieve your symptoms, you don't listen to the consequences.

Getting emphysema, dying of it, the lungs collapsing—these things happen to other people; they don't happen to me. I thought of myself as infallible. I believed that the medicines would keep helping me to feel better; and then, all of sudden, they didn't. My bronchitis got so severe that I couldn't stop coughing. I realized I had to stop smoking.

Having emphysema is scary. It is a downhill ride. You feel that you are ten or fifteen years older than what you actually are. You know that you cannot breathe and that you are dying and that it's happening way too soon. You get up to go to the bathroom and you have a hard time breathing. You want to do things, but you have to have someone there to prepare the way for you. If you go to the grocery store, somebody has to get you a cart so you can put your oxygen tank in it and then you need to lean on the cart as you shop. Someone has to put what you buy in the cart and then carry the groceries inside your home and put them away for you. Somebody has to clean your house, do your dishes, wash your laundry. I have lost interest in just about everything. People like me just sit around waiting to die.

> "I have lost interest in just about everything. People like me just sit around waiting to die."

There is no cure. There is only one thing you can do. If you smoke, quit. If you quit, you can slow down the progression of emphysema, and if you quit early enough, you can even stop it. But if you keep smoking, it is going to eat away at your lungs.

I am on oxygen twenty-four hours a day. I use four liters now; I started out at two liters and that was two years ago. If you have emphysema and you are not getting enough oxygen, cells in your brain are dying. You don't remember things; you can't concentrate.

Quit? I can quit any time. Well, I said that for ten to fifteen years and then found out I was wrong. It was hard. You almost have to kill yourself before you quit. If you are young, in high school, just starting college, and all your friends smoke, you need to get new friends. Don't fall prey to peer pressure. In fact, you should be the peer putting the pressure on others not to smoke. I know kids today say, "You did it when you were a kid; why can't I?" I am trying to tell you that I did it, and I am sorry I did. I wish I never had. I had seen many people with emphysema and on oxygen, and I knew what was coming. But somehow, I managed to tell myself it happened to them; it is not going to happen to me.

Well, it did happen to me. I am not infallible.

What was Bill Andrews's denial story?

Bill's denial story was so entrenched it persisted until he was left with little to gain from stopping smoking. Faced with a choice of smoking or continuing to live, he finally decided to quit using cigarettes. He died not long after his story was written, and I lament that tobacco treatment had not advanced rapidly enough to give him medication options that could have made a difference and helped him to quit sooner.

What is your denial story?

Action steps for people who want to be smoke-free

R.E.C. was fortunate to survive her heart attack, and she used her experience to cement her resolve to remain smoke-free. Some people go through similar experiences and choose to continue smoking. But even a heavy smoker who has a history of heart problems can, with proper treatment and support, become and remain smoke-free. R.E.C.'s and Bill's stories illustrate the importance of knowing your personal denial story. Once you are clear on the story, you are free to examine or question its validity.

Greater self-awareness is one of the benefits of taking up the challenge to become smoke-free. Our thoughts—what we think—are directly connected to our actions—what we do—so knowing what we think can be an important step to changing what we do. R.E.C. used her experience of having a heart attack to change what she was thinking, namely that she smoked so little it couldn't hurt her.

Sue was convinced that smoking just one or two cigarettes a day was fine. In her case, it wasn't a heart attack but rather pressure from her family that got her to quit. Her husband made her understand that smoking made her look and behave in ways she had not seen for herself. And her son made her understand what risk really looks like.

As has already been noted, Bill's great misfortune was that he kept smoking until it was too late to feel much of any benefit from quitting. Once he finally stopped, he regularly attended the Support Group so that his example could motivate others to stop smoking before they, too, became disabled. Sitting in a wheelchair wearing a tube that brought oxygen through his nose, Bill gasped his way through each sentence, describing how smoking had brought him to this point. Sometimes, as he'd pause to catch his breath, he'd have to medicate with several inhalers. His predicament actually moved other smokers to stop while they still had some breath left. And giving back in this way helped Bill to remain smoke-free and kept him from sinking into despair.

Three Key Points

1. Every one of us who smokes has at least one denial story that helps anchor our continued smoking.

2. There is no safe level of smoking. Even an occasional cigarette can put us at risk for relapse and serious health consequences later in life.

3. Becoming aware of a denial story diminishes its power over us.

What is the story you tell yourself that allows you to keep smoking? Take a few minutes to write it down now on the next page. If you did it at the beginning of this chapter, read it again and see if you'd change anything. Ask yourself: *Is it true? What do I get for believing this story? Who would I be without it?*

THE STORY THAT KEEPS ME SMOKING

CHAPTER FOUR

What keeps you tied to smoking?

In our smoking-cessation Groups, we see many smokers who score high on a scale that measures how important they feel it is to stop smoking and how motivated they are to take on the challenge. One way to gauge how important you feel it is to stop smoking is to rate your sense of importance on a scale of zero to ten, with zero being not at all important and ten being extremely important. When we ask this rating question of smokers in our Groups, many respond within the range of seven to ten. With the decision to quit made, they proceed to practice the skills they learn in the program diligently, choose medications, set a quit date, and then embark on a revolving door of stopping and relapsing.

This cycle of quitting and relapsing is not unusual, of course. It speaks to both the recurring nature of the disease and to how addictive cigarettes can be. But sometimes a powerful underlying attachment to cigarettes exists that exerts a pull back to smoking that is much stronger than a person's determination to quit. In such cases, a deeper personal exploration can help to uncover such attachments. There are many ways to engage in this search. Some people turn to psychotherapy; others talk with a trusted friend or mentor. Opening up to your own personal wisdom and analyzing past experiences can also be fruitful. Another way to frame your exploration is to think about why you haven't already quit smoking. Maybe there is something that has worked to hold you back, something that sits in the middle of the road between where you are and the freedom you seek. When you isolate and bring to your attention whatever holds you back, you can set about removing the obstacles to success. Many of these obstacles can be in your external environment (friends who smoke, habit patterns to change, etc.) as well as your internal environment (fear of failure, connections to people with whom you smoked who have now died, etc.)

In this chapter, you will read about two former smokers who, when they uncovered their personal attachment to cigarettes, were finally able to become smoke-free. Looking at what we use smoking to avoid can help uncover what attaches us to it. For example, if we consistently use cigarettes to blunt feelings of sadness, an examination of those feelings, to understand what we are sad about, can loosen the grip of our attachment. We can also ask ourselves questions. For example, What is the worst that could happen to me if I decide to stop smoking? Sometimes the answer is the fear of being a failure. But remember, there are no failures on *this* journey, only lessons. If, for instance, you were learning how to play tennis, there would be plenty of missed balls in the early stages of your practice. By continuing to apply yourself, you would gradually become more proficient. The "mistakes" in life are what give us the chance to learn and develop. They are resources for improvement, especially if we resist the temptation to be self-critical of every missed hit.

Beauty begins the moment you decide to be yourself. **Coco Chanel**

Sandy Bass

Sandy's participation in Group spanned several years. Initially, she attended a complete eight-week series of the cessation program. She then became a regular in the weekly drop-in Group. For months, she would flirt with stopping; she would cut back on the number of cigarettes she smoked and then gradually creep back up to one to two packs a day.

Sandy was like the Group mother, always ready with a kind and understanding word to soothe anyone's feelings. She never raised her voice or became impatient, even when she expressed frustration and despair about her own struggle to overcome dependence on tobacco. And whenever she smoked less, she ate more. She was already overweight, so this pattern became a rationale for her return to smoking. Sandy used nicotine gum sporadically, not really using it enough to change her behavior. She held her denial story about smoking in place by trying just hard enough to support her self-image of being a good person who was trying to change, but not trying hard enough to become successful. If we consistently fall short of our goal

> "If we consistently fall short of our goal to become smoke-free and console ourselves with the message that "at least I'm trying," then this message becomes the denial story that allows us to continue smoking."

to become smoke-free and console ourselves with the message that "at least I'm trying," then this message becomes the denial story that allows us to continue smoking.

Over two years, Sandy became more involved in Group. She managed a phone tree and helped other smokers to stop, while she kept smoking. At the same time that she was becoming a peer counselor, she was also becoming a professional quitter who had yet to stop. After another two or more years had passed, she had gained even more insight and learned even more skills, while she was still stuck. She and I decided to work together privately to see what could be getting in the way of her success.

As we looked into situations and relationships she associated with smoking, Sandy began talking about her best friend—we'll call her Joan—who had been a confidante and companion for years. As Sandy's voice slowed to a whisper, I found myself leaning in to catch what she was saying. She described how she and Joan had given each other a safe haven for exploring and healing the hurts and disappointments in their lives: they commiserated about challenges and shared triumphs. Each shared her innermost life with the other and received the kind of comfort that is special to enduring friendships between women.

For several years, Sandy and Joan volunteered together on a suicide-prevention hotline. Side by side on the telephones, they offered their comfort and wisdom to lonely and suffering souls, all the while smoking one cigarette after another.

Sandy's voice faltered, and it seemed as though her story was winding down; her pace slowed and finally she fell into a long pause. Then, tears that had been welling in the corners of her eyes began to spill over and roll down her cheeks. "What is happening?" I asked her gently. In a barely audible voice, Sandy stuttered: "She died," and then she broke down sobbing. When the heaving of her body finally lessened, her tears, for the moment, spent, I gently inquired what had caused the death of this beloved friend. Sandy's reply jolted through me: "She killed herself."

Was this the event that had prevented Sandy from quitting?

Could it be that smoking had become a way for Sandy to hold on to her dear friend, to shield herself from the finality of her loss? I had to be careful not to impose my perceptions, but when I asked Sandy if she felt any connection between this tragic loss of friendship and her current difficulties with stopping smoking, she confessed feeling that smoking was her last connection to Joan: if she stopped smoking, she would lose her forever.

Many of us experience cigarettes as our friend, even our best friend. For Sandy, this association went deeply into a human relationship. Over the next several days, Sandy and I explored ways for her to keep Joan alive in her memory, to honor her and speak to her in her heart. Soon after, Sandy did stop smoking and the veneer of niceness she had constructed began to crack. She was no longer sweet and kind all the time. She began to express defiance and even anger. Awkward at first, with emotions she had long suppressed or held in check with cigarettes, Sandy began to discover that these so-called darker feelings could be used creatively. A powerful expression of these feelings came with her decision to become an activist in her neighborhood. The Tenderloin is an area of San Francisco with drug-fueled violence. Fed up with the pushers and the crime that thrives around them, Sandy organized her neighbors into reclaiming a multi-block area around their homes. No longer the nice girl, Sandy gathered her anger, took a stand, and announced, "Enough!" Her actions benefited everyone in the neighborhood, and she turned a potential negative—anger—into a real positive—community action.

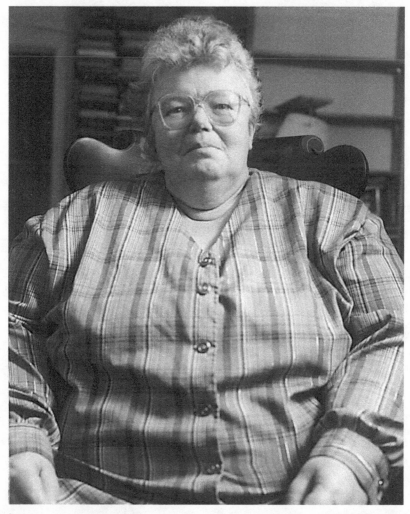

Sandy Bass

Photo by John Harding

Sandy, in Her Own Voice

My smoking expressed a lot of rage and rebelliousness. Both my parents were anti-smokers and anti-drinkers. They spent a lot of time talking about trashy people who smoked and drank, and to annoy them I spent a lot of time trying to be a trashy person who smoked and drank. Thank God I didn't have access to drugs, or I'm sure I would have used them too. I didn't have a feeling that these things would hurt me. In time, I worked myself up to a two-and-a-half-pack-a-day habit.

I did not smoke while I was doing anything else; I always took a break to smoke. I spent an awful lot of time thinking about when I could possibly take a break. I would take a break when I made a mistake or whenever I ran into some problem with what I was doing. Sometimes I wouldn't get back to whatever I had been doing. Now, I finish things. I'm more attuned to the rhythm of something other than my desire for a cigarette, so I get more done, my attention span is greater, and it's easier to focus. Before, there was always a haze or a smokescreen, always something between the world and me.

The only times I stopped smoking were when I was pregnant and when I had major surgery. Had I not had morning sickness, I'm sure I would have smoked when I was pregnant. In general, I told myself, "When it really starts to bother me, I'll quit." I said that through a hacking cough that I couldn't stop. I'd get bronchitis frequently, and I had pneumonia several times, at least two or three times a year.

"Before, there was always a haze or a smokescreen, always something between the world and me."

The Relapse-Prevention Group is vitally important. When I finished the six-week class and I hadn't quit smoking, I would think, "Well, gee, I tried and I couldn't do it." But when you continue coming to a Group, then you can't use that excuse; you have to keep trying until you quit. When I finally did quit smoking, I had been going to the Group for two years; my husband had not smoked for a year and half, and I had done a lot to work up to my quitting. I practiced doing things without a cigarette, like getting up in the morning and not having that first cigarette, not smoking for the first part of the day, or going out to see two movies and coming back in five or six hours without having lit up. At home, I only smoked in the bathroom, and I kept cigarettes where I would have to go through a lot to get one.

Withdrawal from smoking was hard; I felt worse physically than I did when I was recovering from surgery. When you're recovering from surgery, you just accept feeling bad. You know it's going to take time to get better. You know in a week you'll feel a little better, and in a month, you'll really feel better. When I was quitting smoking, I knew that there was something that could make me feel better right away. I knew that all I had to do was walk down to Salem's and fork over a buck seventy-five and I'd have my cigarettes and then I'd feel okay. Knowing I *could* get relief made feeling bad even worse. I had to convince myself I was just going to have to put up with it. The cigarette is not going to help now; I've come too far.

For those first six weeks after I quit for the last time, I was disoriented, confused; I couldn't concentrate at all. I remember getting lost: I got screwed up and got off the bus at the wrong place and I couldn't figure out where I was. It was hard for me to focus. I remember that I was reading and rereading the same book and just not getting anything out of it. I felt emotionally and physically deprived, like I'd lost my second-best friend, if not my best friend. I felt angry and totally unreasonable. I felt like I was back in junior high, which is a time of incredibly strong feelings.

I have arthritis and it was just enhanced; I've never gone through such a bad time. I was using a cane because my legs and feet and knees and hips just felt terrible. I've never used a cane since. When you smoke for 30 years, the change comes on gradually, the bad things, and they also leave gradually, so you have to wait a period of time. Two months after quitting, when I finally started feeling better, I was surprised at how much better I felt.

As a non-smoker, I feel much more powerful, more in control of my life. I have more confidence and I take more chances. Quitting smoking has made me less timid. I now figure, "Well I've done that, so I can do anything." Before, I always felt a sense of dread, like, "Someday you're gonna have to quit smoking and it's gonna be the worst thing you've ever done in your life!" That dread is gone now, so the path ahead is clear. I am freer to think of trying things out. Now, I don't back off of situations and just reach for a cigarette and quiet down. When you don't diffuse your anger, you can focus it where it belongs. I no longer have the feeling that everybody is just gonna run over me. Everything is going better. Once you've done something like quitting smoking, when other things happen, you just don't give up.

> "Two months after quitting, when I finally started feeling better, I was surprised at how much better I felt."

Each of us has our own thing that we do with cigarettes, and our own reasons for why and when we smoke. I felt I could not get through any of the nasty things that life has to offer if I wasn't smoking. The night my daughter was raped, I smoked seven packs of cigarettes. Looking back on it now, what got me through were the people who were doing everything for us, not the smoking. But the first thing I said at the time was that smoking got me through, when, of course, it didn't.

Every once in a while, I will think to myself, "My goodness, I'm not even thinking about smoking! I went through that crisis and it didn't even occur to me to have a cigarette. I did make it without smoking."

What kept Sandy Bass tied to smoking?

Sandy thought smoking protected her and supported her through painful life experiences. In fact, smoking clouded over the power of her feelings and her ability to endure and overcome. Once she quit smoking, she grew into her strength.

I have learned over the years that when one's mind is made up, this diminishes fear; knowing what must be done does away with fear. **Rosa Parks**

Doyle Goodwin

Doyle was born in Louisville, Kentucky, to a Scotch-Irish father and German mother. He went to what he describes as a "really good public school" and, as a young man, he worked as a photographer and writer. While he was growing up, every television show and magazine showed role models with cigarettes.

Doyle started smoking before he was ten years old. By the time he was in his twenties, he was starting to cough. His boss at that time had quit smoking cold turkey two years earlier, and when Doyle asked him how long it took for the desire for a cigarette to leave, his boss replied, "I'll tell you when it happens." His boss's report fueled Doyle's fears about ever stopping smoking. He didn't want to endure that nagging urge and be frustrated and uncomfortable, so he chose to smoke and be frustrated and uncomfortable.

Years later, before he joined Group, Doyle was constantly short of breath; he convinced himself that was a natural state. During a routine medical appointment, he was told he had done permanent damage to his lungs. That news broke through his denial, and he was motivated to find help. He still felt a lot of fear about stopping smoking, not having a clue as to what it or he would be like. We encouraged him to tap in to his years of experience with the 12 steps of Alcoholics Anonymous (AA) and Narcotics Anonymous (NA). Those fellowships had helped him to change his life fundamentally, and he realized that his experience in recovery could be applied to overcoming smoking.

In the process of becoming smoke-free, Doyle understood that to use drugs or cigarettes to change the essential nature of his feelings would not produce any real and lasting change, and that cigarettes, which were the last drugs he was still using, hurt rather than helped him. He further understood that continuing to smoke gave him a handy and self-imposed means of maintaining a poor opinion of himself.

Cutting through the fear that held him tobacco-dependent set Doyle free to deal with more substantive issues, like trying to get along with people and trying to show up, things that he didn't think he could do, just as he thought he couldn't stop smoking.

Another big shift that allowed him to make a radical change was the experience of receiving unconditional love in the recovery program. Up to that time, his experience had often been of people loving him but wanting something in return. Just as in the recovery program in which Doyle got the support to gain sobriety, Group gave him a community of people coming together to do one thing. Joining with others around a common goal helped him to feel stronger and to find the strength that can come from working in a community, rather than suffering in isolation.

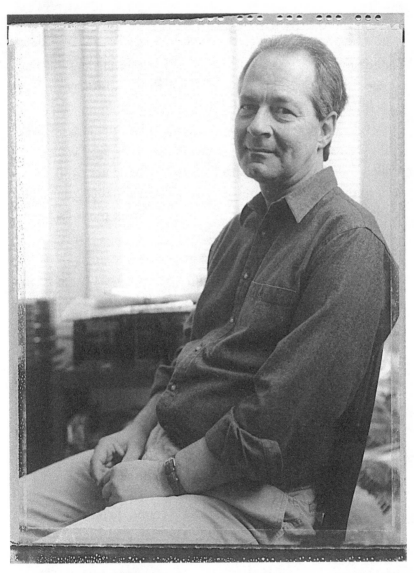

Doyle Goodwin

Photo by John Harding

Doyle Goodwin, in His Own Voice

By the time I was in my mid-twenties, I was a full-time substance abuser, thief, and scofflaw. I didn't know that I didn't have to be an addict. I didn't know that I didn't have to use substances on a daily basis. One of my early heroes was Jean-Paul Sartre, and he always had a cigarette hanging out of his mouth. I thought artists were supposed to suffer and probably die at a young age, and, in the meantime, they were supposed to use all the substances they could. Smoking was one certain way that I could break the rules when I was small; it easily became a habit.

I had been using substances to feel better since I was four years old. After I had my tonsils removed, my folks wouldn't give me any more of the cough syrup that I liked. It was cherry flavored, a pretty red color, and it smelled and tasted good. I would climb up on the back of the toilet and steal it out of the medicine cabinet. Years later I was buying it to go across deserts—a desert being any place that didn't readily sell heroin. The cough syrup made me feel better because it had a lot of codeine in it.

The first active substance abuse I did was when I started smoking. It was the thing to do among my peers. I was seven years old and smoking my mother's Chesterfield Kings. By the time I was in junior high, I was smoking a pack a day. I was always short of breath; I thought that was a natural state. There wasn't a time when I said, "Oh, gee, I can't stop." By the time I actually thought about it, I was hooked. My cigarettes ruled me. Everything I did, even just leaving the house, had me thinking about whether I had enough cigarettes. I'd have done everything, anything to

> "Smoking was one certain way that I could break the rules when I was small; it easily became a habit."

smoke. Even when I didn't have alcohol or heroin, I always had cigarettes.

I used cigarettes to overcome fear, to fit in with friends, or to be hipper or slicker or cooler or whatever it was that I thought I needed to be more of. I thought that I could maybe not use liquor, or not use heroin, but I never thought that I could not use cigarettes. You just smoked until you ended up in your coffin. People didn't stop smoking; fanatics stopped smoking. Normal people just continued to smoke until they died, with a cigarette in their hand.

> "I thought that I could maybe not use liquor, or not use heroin, but I never thought that I could not use cigarettes."

Smoking was part of my nonconformity; it was part of my identification with a class that rebelled. It seemed to be a sign of great mental agitation, and I wanted to think of myself as someone who lived in angst; it went with the creative artist kind of thing. Now I look at people who smoke and think, "How could I have ever thought that was a good thing to do?" I can't remember the process of withdrawal. All of that is overwhelmed by the feeling of joy I have being released from that awful servitude.

In 1991, I did what I had done for years. I got on a 21-day outpatient detox. I wanted to lower my heroin habit so it wasn't so expensive, and I did not want to drink in conjunction with the heroin, because the drinking made my behavior a lot more problematic for me. I wanted to take a rest, build my health back up, and get things under control so that I could use the way I wanted to.

I was really glad to hear someone say, "You know, you can change, you can free yourself." Some people showed me unconditional love, and I had never understood that was actually available in the world. In almost all of the relationships I had ever been in, the message was "If I love you, you owe me." I found out that I could go to AA and NA meetings and I could find other people who were like me who had changed their lives, and maybe I could find a way to change my life. It's very difficult to change unless you're given the ability to change—not made to change, not told that you ought to, but presented with the possibility and then supported as you do it. When I finally got enough unconditional love so that I felt safe, I found the ability to reach out to it and get the help that I needed.

I was nine months clean and sober and smoking three packs a day when I quit using cigarettes. At that time, I was just nuts. If I had a Supplemental Security Income appointment and a General Assistance appointment in the same week, I was overwhelmed. I was terribly threatened by having to go places and do things. I thought everybody I contacted had an attitude, and they did because it was in reaction to my attitude. At one point, I had three appointments in a week, so I just lost my appointment book.

Quitting smoking led into all sorts of situations that I had no idea that it could lead to, one of which is working. I didn't know I could work. I was trying to get on SSI because I didn't want to steal anymore. I wanted to try and lead a somewhat normal life, and I thought probably the best way I could do that was to get SSI and go to meetings. Then I found out that was just the beginning of what I could do. For a long time, I was a thief and a predator and did stuff *to* people to make a living. Now I do stuff *for* people to make a living. That's looking at the world in a whole different way.

Not smoking is a huge help in preventing me from going back to the other substances I once used. I no longer have a single excuse to self-abuse. I don't still smoke and think, "Well, shit, I still smoke, I might as well do this other stuff, too."

I'm able to be part of the solution rather than just disparaging others. My life is a lot different. The last capstone to the fountain of ability and freedom was removed. I don't have to be the guy standing outside the doorway, hunched over in the rain, puffing on a cigarette. I don't have to worry about where, what, and how I'm going to smoke.

I know now that relief doesn't come from outside you. You can't take something and have things really change or really be better. I've learned it's okay to be uncomfortable. I don't have to take all those feelings as seriously as I once thought I did. And I don't have to fix them. I just go, "Oh, that's just that crazy part, and it'll be gone in a little while or a longer while, whenever it is." It's a gift that I never thought that I'd get.

What kept Doyle Goodwin tied to smoking?

Until he quit smoking, Doyle had assumed he needed cigarettes to fix whatever felt uncomfortable or unbearable. He needed to have something to rely on that didn't ask for anything in return. After he quit, he woke up to the knowledge that cigarettes had taken a lot from him and he could rely on himself, he was whole, and he was okay without cigarettes.

What keeps you tied to smoking?

Action steps for people who want to be smoke-free

Our relationship with cigarettes usually has many layers, including the physical consequences of addiction and withdrawal and the effect of inhaled nicotine on our emotional life. The repetitive nature of self-medicating through cigarettes reinforces emotional patterns and dependencies. If many of the cigarettes we smoke shield us from unpleasant emotional states by releasing pleasant and reinforcing chemicals in our brains, we unwittingly create the sense that whatever we are hiding is more than we could handle, should it be revealed. In short, we teach ourselves that we cannot face our fears; each cigarette reinforces the belief that we are weaker than we may actually be.

On the surface, Sandy seemed like an ordinary person, but stopping smoking brought out the hero in her. When she finally gave up cigarettes, something in her was unblocked that allowed her to impact her whole community in a positive way. Think about it: what could your smoking be blocking that, once released, will make your world a better place?

Stopping smoking is usually about a lot more than stopping smoking. Becoming free of cigarettes, we have the opportunity to let go of negative thoughts that hold us back from personal development. For many of us, these thoughts have to do with our sense of self-worth and self-acceptance. Doyle's story illustrates a

> Think about it: what could your smoking be blocking that, once released, will make your world a better place?

relatively common phenomenon: a lack of experience with being loved or feeling lovable. When we don't love ourselves, when we are critical and mean and self-deprecating, it's hard to muster the energy to make positive changes in our lives. This is one place where Group experiences can be tremendously healing. Doyle found that being in a community that cared about him gave him the basis to translate that caring into doing something difficult and healthy: stopping smoking.

As smokers, we are used as a revenue source for the tobacco industry. We are bombarded with messages suggesting that smoking will give us relief from a lack of self-worth. For example, the early Virginia Slims campaign played on women's desire to be thin. Ads for Benson & Hedges suggested that smokers would enjoy an aura of success and abundance. Adolescents are encouraged to smoke, through messages that portray smoking as an adult decision. What better way to prey on a teenager's desire to be perceived as grown-up and mature than to say smoking is for adults?

Taking an unflinching look at ourselves to see where we might feel inadequate or vulnerable takes courage. Try asking yourself a few questions: *What feelings does smoking help me to avoid? When I think about stopping smoking, what feelings come up? If one of those feelings is fear, what is the worst that could happen? Do I deserve to be happy and successful? What were some of my early motivations to start smoking?*

Years ago, you might have started smoking to be part of a peer group. Today, what might you do to give yourself an experience of belonging? Perhaps joining a stop-smoking program would be a good first step. If you started smoking to look cool or sexy, how else might you cultivate that look today? Or, if you felt you needed to smoke to be interesting and desirable, what activities could you cultivate today that would help to make you a more fascinating and appealing person?

> Today, what might you do to give yourself an experience of belonging?

Three Key Points

1. As long as we think we need cigarettes to get by in life, we can't see that we've got what we need within ourselves without relying on tobacco.

2. Opening ourselves to look underneath our fears can reveal strengths and capacities that are life-enhancing and changing.

3. To get free of tobacco's hold on us, we must summon courage to feel and do what we've used cigarettes to avoid.

NOTES

_____

_____

_____

_____

_____

_____

_____

_____

_____

_____

_____

_____

_____

_____

_____

_____

_____

_____

_____

_____

_____

CHAPTER FIVE

I'm already sick, so what's the difference if I smoke?

Combating the negative effects of cigarettes is a drain on the body's resources. That means that many illnesses are only made worse by smoking. In addition, some medications used to treat chronic disease are not as effective when we smoke. For example, people being treated for high blood pressure may need higher doses of their prescription. Likewise, patients being treated for diabetes might need higher doses of insulin. A smoker with diabetes will have a higher risk for amputation than someone with diabetes who does not smoke.

Information about the relationship between smoking and the recurrence of certain cancers is sobering. Breast cancer survivors have a greater risk of recurrence if they smoke. Even a person with lung cancer, one of the most frightening possibilities facing smokers, will tolerate his or her treatments better and face better outcomes by stopping smoking. Each of the women in this chapter has medical problems that are made worse by smoking. Because they believed that they could not recover from the illnesses that already plagued them, they questioned the value of stopping smoking.

For him who has conquered the mind, the mind is the best of friends; but for one who has failed to do so, his mind will remain the greatest enemy.
Buddha

Joyce Lavey

Joyce attended the stop-smoking program for more than two years before she successfully stopped smoking. A highly intelligent woman with an air of angry defiance, she was worn down by family hardships and illnesses. She herself had survived breast cancer and had sisters who had died from lung cancer and other tobacco-related diseases. Like many smokers, Joyce could be merciless in her self-judgment regarding her behavior and what she thought her smoking meant about her as a person. Cigarettes gave her a handy excuse for seeing herself in a negative light. She managed to put herself in a class of her own, even in the cessation-support Group. No one was as "stupid" as she was for smoking—"I'm a cancer survivor, for God's sake!"—and no one, in her estimation, was less likely to become a non-smoker. Joyce had so much sadness in her life that it hung on her like a heavy coat.

She was the most surprised of anyone when she did finally quit smoking. A new optimism and energy started to emerge, and she began to get more involved in life. As she became more sociable and outgoing, she found she was able to experience happiness. Stopping smoking removed a serious risk factor for cancer recurrence and gave her the satisfaction of feeling self-confident and self-caring.

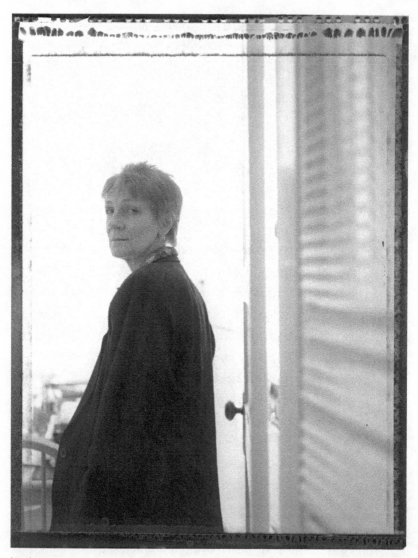

Joyce Lavey   Photo by John Harding

Joyce Lavey, in Her Own Voice

One day when my parents were gone and my sister and I were taking care of their grocery store, I took a pack of cigarettes and said, "I'm gonna smoke." It was sort of a fuck-you thing to my parents. My mother's reaction was, "Nyaa nyaa nyaa, well you think you're so smart smoking," so I lit up another one.

I was going away to college and I couldn't afford to eat three meals [a day], so I smoked and ate just one meal. It helped me to manage not knowing if I was going to make it financially or otherwise. I used smoking to manage feelings of anger, fear, and sadness.

When I was angry at somebody I would sit and think about how I was going to express my anger to them. I would always think with my cigarettes, and after one, I might have another to think even more. For 25 years, I was really angry with myself that I ever started. I was very anti-smoking before I ever smoked, and I never ever imagined I would get hooked. I didn't like being addicted.

I mentally worked at quitting, but I didn't make many real attempts to quit, for 29 years. Before I quit, I went to Nicotine Anonymous (NA) for two and a half years. There, I didn't attempt to quit smoking. I just wanted to keep it at the same level. I was finally pushed over the edge because my oldest sister was diagnosed with terminal lung cancer and that scared the shit out of me. I had been diagnosed with breast cancer myself a few years earlier and I was still smoking.

There is a gene factor in my family for breast cancer. For the four years I smoked after my diagnosis, I would say to myself, "I wish I had quit. Maybe I could have prevented this." When I was diagnosed, I thought I'd be gone before my siblings. I never would've thought that seven years later two sisters would have died, one of lung cancer, the other of a pulmonary embolism; another sister would be diagnosed with lung cancer and have a lung removed; and still another one would have lung cancer and be getting chemo. My brother still smokes. I thought, "The best I can do is to put myself in Groups and talk about it."

People I knew in Nicotine Anonymous and Group were supportive of me, for two and a half years. They never made fun of me for coming even though I was smoking. They kept nagging me about a quit date, so, to satisfy them, I picked a date, but I never intended to follow through. The day came, and I didn't have a whole lot riding on it. I didn't say "If you quit, you're good. If you don't, you're bad." I put the patch on and that was it. It worked, and I never expected it to. I never, ever thought I would quit smoking.

I spent so many years whipping myself about not being able to quit that I got to the point where I gave up punishing myself. When I gave up, it allowed space for some kind of strength that I didn't even know existed.

> "I spent so many years whipping myself about not being able to quit that I got to the point where I gave up punishing myself."

Not being so hard on yourself is a good start. When I was always at myself, I was putting myself in a weakened position.

The nicotine patch really helped. I had temper tantrums, but it wasn't like I had imagined it would be. The thing that kept me from quitting smoking all those years was that I didn't want to experience the extreme discomfort of going through withdrawal, and I didn't want to gain weight. I only gained a few pounds. I started running, and I went to the movies practically every night for the first two to three weeks. I bought a pacifier, so when I got really uptight, I would chew on the pacifier. I had a lot of trouble carrying on conversations with people, especially if they bored me or they were long-winded. I just wanted to shut 'em up.

After stopping smoking, I got in touch with lots of anger. I found that I could track it more easily because I didn't have a distraction. I also got in touch with how sad I was. I always knew that, but I didn't know it went

> "Just because you smoked three or five cigarettes doesn't mean you can't put the patch back on and start all over again."

that deep. The turning point was finding out that one of my favorite sisters was dying. That brought it right home, bang! Even breast cancer didn't bring it home to me; her death brought it home to me.

I'm angry at all the death and illness. I have begun feeling the pain, and when it hits, it's like a ton of bricks, like my heart is just breaking. What surprised me in quitting smoking was that I was able to experience the death of my sister and my father's death and then another sister's death, all of this really heavy stuff, without returning to smoking. I wonder if I could have done that if I hadn't been chewing Nicorette gum.

One sister had tried a number of times to quit and had not been successful, but she was very supportive of me. When I relapsed, she said, "Just because you smoked three or five cigarettes doesn't mean you can't put the patch back on and start all over again." She really helped me quit.

Cigarettes helped me isolate. Now, there isn't that barrier, so I relate to people. When I smoked, I could distance myself with cigarettes. I could stay home with cigarettes rather than seek company. Now I turn to people for support more than in the past. I'm more genuine, more honest with people, and honest with myself about what my needs are and what I want. I'm a kinder person, more considerate, and more generous than I was before. I'm more even tempered, I flare up less, and I'm more tolerant. I don't have all that shame I had about smoking. I don't have that mental agony, that torture. I feel so much better.

My self-esteem is higher, and I feel more attractive. I feel able to handle most things in my life because I'm doing it without cigarettes. I thought I was strong before. But now I realize I have an amazing amount of strength that I didn't even know I had. When I was a smoker, I felt very weak. I felt all my strength was false because I was dependent. Now, I'm the one who's sitting inside myself. I am more real and more vulnerable and less interested in maintaining an image. I value myself and my life over smoking.

I now see how people sacrifice their health and well-being to cigarettes. The tobacco companies disgust me. I believe in people's right to smoke. But having one sister die at 61, another sister lose a lung at 52, and still another sister with stage three lung cancer at 52, I see it's a human sacrifice, and it's very sad. I don't condemn people for smoking, I just feel sad because of my own experience.

I was so grateful to quit smoking after 29 years. I never thought I would be able to do it. I thought I was married to cigarettes—that I was in a prison serving a sentence. Why would I want to go back to all that self-hatred that comes with smoking? Life is rough enough without that torture. Here I was with breast cancer and I was smoking. I hated myself every time I lit a cigarette and always said to myself, "Who is this person? She must want to die." That self-torture is what I didn't want to return to.

I felt like a hard-core, I'll-die-with-a-cigarette-in-my-hand person. No matter how hopeless people feel, they should never give up. I am a testament to hopelessness turned hopeful.

I'm already sick, so what's the difference if I smoke?

Much of Joyce's daily life was darkened by the facts of her own and her family's poor health. Cancer infused her life with both cynicism—she did not see why she should bother to quit—and despair—if she did quit, it wouldn't make any difference. Quitting smoking led her to feel more optimistic and cheerful in her life and increased her chances of a good prognosis against cancer.

Then comes a moment of feeling the wings you've grown, lifting. **Rumi**

Chauncey McLorin

Chauncey, a young single mother, started smoking before she was diagnosed with a chronic disease. Cheerful, friendly, and outgoing, Chauncey added humor and light-heartedness to the smoking-cessation Group. She usually brought her young daughter, Danina, along with her, and the love and care the two shared was obvious and heartwarming. Danina, who was somewhat shy and who would quietly entertain herself while the Group met, made it abundantly clear that she wanted her mom to stop smoking.

Chauncey suffers from sarcoidosis, a chronic disease with no known cure that creates fibrous tissue most often in the lungs. Given that smoking directly attacks the lungs, continuing to smoke had a devastating impact on Chauncey's well-being. One of the reasons she smoked, however, was to give herself emotional comfort from the hopelessness of her disease. Even though she was very young, her smoking robbed her of so much energy that she felt like an old person. Her recovery from tobacco dependence had such a dramatic effect that everyone in the Group was aware of the difference in her. Chauncey modeled the benefits of quitting and she had a powerful role in motivating others to follow her lead.

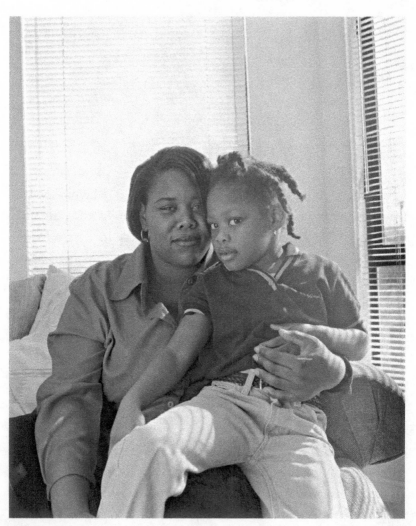

Chauncey McLorin

Photo by John Harding

Chauncey McLorin, in Her Own Voice

I was born in San Francisco. I have three sisters and one brother. My brother, one sister, my mom, my grandmother, and my dad all smoke.

When I was thirteen, I would steal cigarettes. Then I got caught. My mom bought a pack, and I had taken a few out of it. She said, "I just bought this pack. Why is it gone already?" As soon as she left, I went into the bathroom and started smoking. She came right back and there I was, puffing away. She asked me "Do you smoke?" and I said, "Yeah." She said "Don't smoke outside. You can smoke in the house." I thought I was going to be killed, but she didn't get mad, so that was like permission to go for it. Every now and then, she would bring me a pack. That was terrible; I wish she would have just told me not to smoke.

Everybody was smoking. My little sisters were smoking with me. I was a bad influence. Cigarettes were 75 cents a pack. My friends and I would get together and walk to school, rather than use our bus fare. When we'd get up enough change, we'd buy some cigarettes and smoke. I thought I was grown-up with a cigarette in my hand, but I was still a child.

Once I mastered inhaling and blowing the smoke out my nose, I was smoking full blast, two packs a day, one cigarette after the other. If I didn't get that last hit, and the cigarette burned out, I'd smoke a whole other one. If the cigarette went out by itself, I'd get another one and work on that.

I started losing weight. I couldn't eat; I was just shriveling. I slept all the time and I could barely get out the bed. When I'd walk, I needed assistance. It got really bad. I felt like somebody real elderly. I was so sick. My sickness didn't come on slowly. It came on fast. One day I was all right, the next I was not all right, and I was still trying to smoke. I was smoking the lightest cigarette on the market and it still burned my throat. I coughed so hard that I couldn't talk. [I was] scared to death.

I found out that I had sarcoidosis. I started on medication. I couldn't breathe, and I was still smoking. Cigarettes were going to be the death of me. I said, "I can't take it no more, I have to stop to stay alive." The only thing I could think of was staying alive. Going through the program and listening to other people's experiences helped a lot.

By stopping smoking and saving my own life, I'm not hurting anybody anymore. Not smoking, not hurting my child, makes me a better parent. Your kids are a product of you. If your parents smoke, you grow up to smoke. If my daughter sees me smoking, she'll want to smoke.

> "If your parents smoke, you grow up to smoke. If my daughter sees me smoking, she'll want to smoke."

I need to learn how to help the children. I don't like Danina to be around cigarette smoke, so no smoking in here. I talk to her and tell her all the bad things that happened to me when I was smoking, almost dying. I tell her that my serious cigarette smoking contributed to my lung disease—that it made it much worse, to the point that she almost wouldn't have been born.

Last year, I smoked for a month or two. I was going out to parties, and when I'd have a drink, I'd want to have a cigarette. That's how I started again. Before I knew it, I was buying packs of cigarettes. I started smoking just on the weekend, then it was every day. And then, one day, I started coughing. Danina said, "Why are you smoking those cigarettes?" She would be picking at the butts in the ashtray, playing with them, and that really turned me off. I quit because of that.

Once I got over the first few days, I was okay, but man it was hard. Cigarettes, they pull you in. Your body is telling you that you need just one more, and then you have to resist it, so that's the hard part the first few days. Once that was over, I was okay. I could smell fresh air, and I just kept occupied.

I go to functions now, and if there's alcohol, I don't even bother, because I like to be in my right mind. Alcohol and drugs and all that stuff impair you so that you can't protect yourself. That's why I stay away from that type of thing.

I had to keep in my mind that this was what I really want to do, and I did. I didn't want to be smoking around my daughter, burning holes in everything. I said to myself that "This has to stop; it just has to stop. I don't want to smoke, and I don't talk to nobody who smokes. And that might be the man of my dreams, but if he smokes, I'm passing him up. I don't want to smoke, and as long as I keep saying that, I'll be all right."

I felt good about myself being able to conquer the cigarette. I'm healthier because I am not smoking. My child is healthier because I am not smoking around her. I feel good about myself because I'm not hurting anybody anymore.

A lot of people that I talk to say that they only smoke cigarettes. I say cigarettes kill, just like drugs and alcohol.

I'm already sick, so what's the difference if I smoke?

The combination of sarcoidosis and smoking left Chauncey feeling like an old woman. She barely had enough energy to care for herself, much less for her young daughter. By stopping smoking, Chauncey got her life back and she was able to be a proud young mother.

I am not discouraged because every wrong attempt discarded is another step forward.
Thomas Alva Edison

Linda McNicoll

The last story in this chapter belongs to Linda. A jolly, cheerful, and thoughtful person, Linda could no longer work as a registered nurse because of complications from diabetes. She was eager to stop smoking and maintain the health she had left. She was also motivated because her young nieces were very anxious about what smoking was doing to their beloved auntie. Linda approached stopping smoking in an organized, practical, and methodical manner, much as, I imagined, she had practiced nursing.

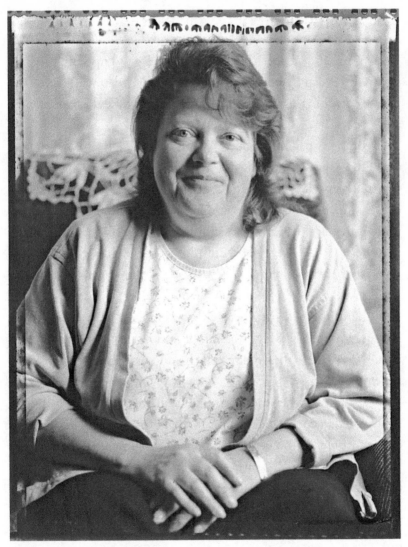

Linda McNicoll

Photo by Greene and Harding

Linda McNicoll, in Her Own Voice

I was born and raised in San Francisco. I grew up living in this house. I went to school around the corner. My dad worked for the phone company; my mom cut mattresses. I worked as a nurse for a few years.

Both my parents smoked. When I got to high school, I started smoking. Like typical kids do, I sneaked my parents' cigarettes. I was up to a pack a day in high school. I felt like it was cool because of the kids. I would come home from school and blow the smoke up the fireplace. I didn't smoke in front of my parents until I was in college. I felt that they would be disappointed in me if they knew that I was smoking. I spent my childhood trying to be the perfect kid.

If I didn't tell the doctors that I smoked; they never knew. Because my chest was always clear, I didn't have symptoms that you usually associate with smoking. If the doctors asked if I smoked, I never denied it.

It didn't bother me to smoke until we all became aware of what smoking could do to people. When I was working in intensive care, I would go on a break and return—smelling of cigarette smoke—to my patients on respirators. Where was my head? I was in complete denial. I remember one lady who had bad asthma and emphysema. She had smoked as a younger person and was in the intensive-care unit every two months. She was 82 years old and no bigger than a peanut. I would take care of her, and then go on my break and have my cigarette.

Over the years, smoking just lost its appeal. I would smoke, and it wouldn't taste good. I would be chain-smoking and I would ask myself, "Why am I doing this?" I would wake up and my mouth would feel like barefoot soldiers had been marching through it. I wasn't enjoying it, but I didn't have the *oomph* to stop.

I got sick. I didn't know I had diabetes, and it reached the point where I couldn't work. I had increasing problems, with my leg

"I wasn't enjoying it, but I didn't have the *oomph* to stop."

getting weak. My eye doctor picked up on the eye changes. I still have a lot of nerve damage in my legs, tingling in my fingers, and problems with poor eyesight.

I would spend most of my time in the living room. My nieces were starting to rag on me about smoking. They live here in this house. One of them has asthma pretty bad; she has been hospitalized a couple of times. I felt guilty smoking around them. I knew it wasn't good for them.

Because of the neuropathy in my leg, I wasn't too mobile. I know that smoking causes circulatory problems. I figured that if I stopped smoking, some of the problems with my leg might improve. My toes and feet were numb, and I just didn't need the added cardiac problems. That's the big thing with diabetes: cardiac problems can develop.

When I started going to the smoking-cessation classes, I was up to two and a half packs a day. I was beginning to feel it, and I realized that with the diabetes, I did not need the additional stress and problems that cigarette smoking causes. I had been coughing, had been thinking about quitting, and when the doctor suggested smoking cessation, I figured I would give it a try.

My sister and my brother-in-law both smoke. And they live here. I depend on my sister to drive me places. When I was quitting, I had no way of getting to a store to buy cigarettes, and she refused to buy them for me. She was keeping her cigarettes downstairs so that I could not get to them. I was irritable when I quit, but I didn't try and force her to give me one. I was determined. Now, they will smoke in front of me. It didn't bother me when I first stopped, but the last six, eight months, the cigarette smoke gets to me. It irritates me—yuck.

I was having lots of problems because of the neuropathy. A big motivator to quit smoking was a chance that it could improve the sensations in my feet and my hands, in part because I like to do stitchery. Everything just kind of came together and gave me the courage and the willpower to say, "Okay, I will stop."

I knew that it was going to be hard, but it wasn't as hard as I thought it was going to be. I thought it was going to be impossible. I thought I was going to be jittery and that I would put on weight. I didn't want to do that. I would have cravings and I was irritable, but I wasn't out of control. Deep breathing and drinking lots of water helped.

My nieces and my sister did a lot of stroking. They would say, "Great work, Auntie: one more day, one more day." They were very positive.

I am coming up on my two-year anniversary, and I hate what would have been going on if I had been smoking for these last two years. I don't get as short of breath as I did. I don't cough or have the respiratory problems that I did. My legs would not be as good as they are. I can control my diabetes a lot better. My stamina has improved. I am more active now than I was. I am out there with my visor hat and my wrap-around sunglasses, walking. When I smoked, I could not climb the stairs without help. But now I can climb the stairs on my own.

Doctors need to let their patients know what the options are. Letting me know that the smoking-cessation clinic was available but not belittling me and making me feel like an imbecile for smoking was important to me. It made me feel like it was my decision to go there if I wanted to do it.

> "I played a lot of video games to get through those periods. It kept my fingers and my mind occupied."

The hardest times were after that morning cup of coffee and after dinner. I played a lot of video games to get through those periods. It kept my fingers and my mind occupied. I would play in the girls' room. That was my safe zone. I was not going to smoke there. And then I was not going to smoke in the dining room, where we eat. I was not going to sit in there after dinner and smoke, so I narrowed it down.

I didn't have any place where I was going to smoke. It just wasn't worthwhile to get up and stand on the porch. I stopped, and I am proud of myself for quitting. I really achieved something important that is good for me and makes my nieces feel good about me. They used to complain that my breath would always stink. My gums are messed up because of the diabetes and smoking. I had major gum surgery.

I used to see cigarettes and I would think, "Oh, just one wouldn't hurt," but I have reached the point where it is really not worth it to me. I won't take the chance of getting hooked on cigarettes now because I don't want to go through it all again. Smoking is not cool, and it is not good for me. With all my other medical problems, it is not safe for me. It is just not worth the hassle.

Quitting wasn't as hard as I thought it was going to be. The most important thing was I did not have access to cigarettes. My sister would not let me near hers. She really loves me. It makes a difference to have that support. I had to deal with it just like I had to deal with my diabetes. You are not going to smoke. You cannot have cigarettes, so deal with it.

If you have the urge to stop smoking, go with it. It is really important, and you will feel really good about yourself when you do it. It is a big accomplishment.

I'm already sick, so what's the difference if I smoke?

Linda had a lot to lose by smoking. Her mobility and vision had already been affected by diabetes. When she stopped smoking, she was able to regain some of her independence and no longer required assistance for things like climbing the stairs to her home.

I'm already sick, so what's the difference if I smoke?

Action steps for people who want to be smoke-free

If you're already feeling ill, it can be challenging to muster the resources to stop smoking. Chronic illness typically takes a toll on a person's physical and emotional life. Having to live with the stress and uncertainty of poor health can make it difficult to enjoy life and to feel positive emotions. A general negativity starts to drain your energy and ability to feel happy. When smoking is added to the equation, you have a handy tool for magnifying all kinds of bad feelings, including hopelessness.

On the other hand, we all know people who endure terrible things with a bright and positive demeanor. But the additional strain put on the body from smoking can be enough to tip the balance into the negative, which means that stopping smoking can improve how a person feels about life in general. This shift of feeling can be seen in Joyce's story: as her anger dissipated, she became more self-confident and connected with others. She was also able to enjoy knowing that stopping smoking had reduced the risk of a recurrence of her cancer.

When Joyce felt pressured by other people to change, that pressure added to the pressure she was already putting on herself. In reaction to feeling pressured, many of us smoke. Cigarettes muffle the uncomfortable feeling that pressure provokes. Pressure from within ourselves can have the same effect. For months, Joyce played at the edges of becoming a non-smoker; it wasn't until she spontaneously decided to set a quit date that she was surprisingly (to her) successful.

Are you someone who does well under pressure? Does setting goals help you progress, or does it fuel a sense of inadequacy? One of our Group participants allowed himself to smoke any four days of a week. He went along for several months, planning his life around those four days, until one day he was fed up

> "How do you look at stopping smoking? Is there a way in which you are taking it so seriously that it feels almost impossible to achieve?"

with that effort and decided to go for it and stop smoking. That tactic was related to Joyce's decision to placate her peers in NA by choosing a quit date, and then on that day, without any pressure, she put on the patch and quit.

Stopping smoking is an extremely important decision. In fact, it is *the* most important thing we can do for our health. In other words, it really matters. And it can especially matter in people who are already sick. At the same time, *making* a big deal of it can become an obstacle to success. What often becomes magnified is what we feel we're losing, rather than the relief and benefits we can ultimately enjoy. How do you look at stopping smoking? Is there a way in which you are taking it so seriously that it feels almost impossible to achieve? How could you take some of the pressure off of yourself and approach the challenge more playfully? One woman we worked with had cancer and was going to need surgery in a week. Her doctor told her she must quit smoking before the surgery. She called us in a panic: she had never had a smoke-free day in 43 years of smoking. We talked for half an hour, giving her room to report her smoking history and explore all she liked and didn't like about smoking. Then we suggested that she tell herself she was *stopping for the surgery*, not *quitting*. She could decide about quitting later. This made the goal reachable, and after the surgery, she worked on staying smoke free.

You can experiment with ways to postpone or cut down on cigarettes without actually committing to quitting. For example, try distracting yourself from smoking in habitual situations. Or, make a bet with yourself: "I bet I can go X hours without a cigarette." When the urge arises, remind yourself you have only a little more time to go to win your bet. Be sure to reward yourself when you win.

Changing elements of your smoking rituals is another way to get playful with your process. Open your cigarette pack from the bottom. If you usually hold your cigarette in your right hand, hold it in your left. Or try placing your cigarette between your pinkie and ring fingers.

Smokers with chronic illnesses usually feel at least some relief from their symptoms fairly quickly after stopping. Focusing on that relief and being as aware as possible of the contrast between how you felt as a smoker and now as a non-smoker can help keep you going through the hard times. Take a moment here and think about any symptoms you have that either came from or were made worse by smoking. What are those symptoms? How do they affect the quality of your life? What will you enjoy more by being smoke-free?

In as much detail as possible, think about what feeling better would be like. Would you have more energy? Would you breathe more easily? Would you be free of bronchitis or frequent colds? Would you worry less about how your health is being impacted and what the future might be for you? Take a few minutes and jot down some of those details here. Then, if you feel ready, also note some first steps you might take to bring you closer to feeling those improvements in your life.

> What would you enjoy about being smoke-free? In as much detail as possible, think about what feeling better would be like. Take a few minutes and jot down some of those details on the notes page.

Linda knew the toll that cigarettes were taking on her health and how they worsened the effect of her diabetes. She was fearful of losing her ability to walk and care for herself and of losing her independence. She used that fear constructively to ignite her determination to protect the abilities she had by making specific plans to move herself to becoming a non-smoker. She also had a skill that is key to closing down the revolving door that leads back to smoking: she was aware of her limits. Knowing that exposure to cigarettes would put her at risk, she put them out of her reach. She did not play the game of *I should be able to resist cigarettes* by testing herself and keeping them around. She also knew to stay busy, occupying both her fingers and her mind to keep herself away from the behavior she was changing.

What are your limits? What are your irresistible temptations to smoke? What are some triggers that you could temporarily remove from your life, such as lunch breaks with smoking friends or a particular walk during which you have a cigarette?

What are some things you could do to keep yourself busy and distracted? Could knitting or drawing or cooking engage you happily? If, like Chauncey and Linda, there are children in your life, getting into your playful side by hanging out with them could help support you through the first weeks and months.

Three Key Points

1. Any chronic disease is made worse by smoking, even to the point of requiring amputation or open-heart surgery.

2. Stopping smoking removes a huge burden from the body and allows it to use resources and reserves for healing.

3. Quitting smoking may result in needing less medication to treat chronic conditions.

NOTES

_____

_____

_____

_____

_____

_____

_____

_____

_____

_____

_____

_____

_____

_____

_____

_____

_____

_____

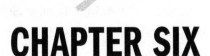

CHAPTER SIX

Who besides you is affected by your smoking, and how would they benefit if you stopped?

If you are a smoker who lives with children and/or pets and you go outside to smoke, that is good news. Why good news, you ask? First, for your own benefit, going outside means you are putting a limit on where you smoke, indicating some choice and control over your behavior. And second, eliminating second- and third-hand smoke exposure in your home makes a difference to everyone's health. So if this is something you've always held to or if it is a new decision, congratulations.

An estimated 38,112 lung cancer and heart disease deaths annually are attributable to exposure to second-hand smoke. We have only begun to explore the effects of a new category called third-hand smoke, the residue that is left on the clothing and hair of the smoker and in carpets and drapes in areas where people smoke. Cotinine is a byproduct of nicotine metabolism, and the more you smoke, the higher your blood or urine levels of cotinine will be. Cotinine levels are detected in the urine of infants who crawl in rooms where there has been smoking. My personal concern as a smoker was that I was not only modeling behavior I did not want my child to mimic, I was also exposing her to toxins that were bad for her health.

One of the most gratifying rewards of working as a Certified Tobacco Treatment Specialist (CTTS) comes when the benefits of quitting spread to include more people than the smokers themselves. When a pregnant woman shows up to class, we are excited for the opportunity to support the well-being of both the mother and unborn child. Caroline, a young African-American woman, comes immediately to mind. Twenty-eight years old, she had been smoking since she was twelve and had always planned to stop before trying to get pregnant. Faced with an unplanned pregnancy, she was desperate to stop smoking and was wrestling with terrible guilt because, by the end of her first trimester, she had not yet quit.

We had two or three phone calls with Caroline before she decided to join the program. She was hesitant to join Group as she expected the others to judge her as she judged herself. As it turned out, the Group in which she enrolled also included Melinda, an older woman who, five weeks prior, had been diagnosed with lung cancer and had not stopped smoking even though she knew her medical treatments would be more effective if she quit. Melinda, like Caroline, was scared about exposing herself to judgment from the Group.

Especially because of the intensity of their predicaments, having Caroline and Melinda in the same Group actually inspired an immediate deepening of bonds among *all* the participants. Everyone was struck with the realization that tobacco is powerfully addictive and that most smokers require treatment with medications and counseling to overcome its hold.

Caroline's first hurdle in overcoming smoking was to deal with self-judgment. Learning to separate her self-value from the smoking behavior, she began to understand that she was dealing with a chronic disease—and that the difficulties she was experiencing said more about the disease than they did about her. Her love and concern for her unborn child motivated her to get the upper hand on smoking. In addition to working on changing her thoughts and behavior, Caroline chose to use medication, and she did, in fact, become smoke-free. When her beautiful and healthy baby boy was born, she brought him to Group and we thanked him for helping to save his mother's life. By stopping smoking, she was ensuring a longer and healthier life than she could have enjoyed as a smoker, and in loving her son in this way, she was giving him a gift of health that might otherwise have been taken away.

Whether you think you can or you think you can't, you're right. Henry Ford

Marsha Akins and Jerome Davis

In the pages that follow, you will read about Marsha and Jerome, a young couple living with their three daughters. When I went to interview them, the two youngest girls were at home and their lively play punctuated our conversation.

Jerome was the first of the two parents to enroll in Group. I remember looking up to see a tall, gangly man standing in the doorway. He wore a wool cap and leather jacket even though the day was warm. Accompanying him were two little girls who were obviously well cared for even though they coughed throughout the meeting and their noses ran steadily. Jerome straight off admitted to being afraid he could not quit; he had tried many times over the years and had always gone back to smoking. His family had suffered multiple deaths from various cancers, and he was terrified that his own smoking would lead to cancer and a terrible death.

After stopping smoking, Jerome came regularly to the weekly drop-in Relapse-Prevention Support Group, always with the two little girls. One evening, he arrived with a beautiful young woman who, I soon learned, was the girls' mother. Marsha was in drug recovery and had met Jerome while she was pregnant with the youngest of her three daughters.

Marsha entered a drug treatment program and became clean and sober. Jerome went to parenting classes and, with his support,

Marsha was eventually able to take back her two older daughters from foster care. The two adults and three girls became a family.

As Jerome went through the process of stopping smoking, Marsha watched him very carefully. A heavy smoker herself, she had enjoyed having him as her smoking buddy and was uncomfortable with Jerome's decision to quit. He, however, was not to be deterred. Frightened about so many of his relatives' having died from cancer, Jerome wanted to do whatever he could to decrease his risk factors.

After each stop-smoking meeting, Jerome went home and shared what he learned with Marsha. In the weeks leading up to his quit date, he began to smoke only outside in the yard, explaining to Marsha that the hazards of second-hand smoke were putting their daughters at risk. In fact, the little girls had been getting nebulizer-breathing treatments for asthma symptoms several times a day. Jerome told Marsha that exposure to smoke was particularly bad for people with asthma. Soon, both parents began to smoke only outside of the house.

Marsha continued to watch Jerome's process almost (she admitted to this) hoping that he would be unsuccessful, so she wouldn't have to live with a non-smoker. She was afraid he *would* quit, because then *she* would feel less comfortable as a smoker, and she thought she'd rather keep smoking. But Jerome kept plugging along, and soon he was building up weeks and months as a non-smoker. He was a regular participant in the Relapse-Prevention Support Group, benefitting from both the support he got and what he gave. His self-esteem as a successful quitter made him that much more determined not to turn back.

Jerome would still show up to Group with the two girls, who played happily and quietly while their step-dad participated in the nonsmoking community. Then one evening, Marsha showed up, too. She stayed in the back of the room, observing but not participating in the discussions. As the weeks went by, she gradually began to share her own story, as she began to seriously consider taking on the challenge of becoming smoke-free.

In time, that was her decision, and you will read in her story of the success she achieved. Within a few weeks of both parents becoming smoke-free, their daughters stopped needing nebulizer treatments for their asthma. As is often the case in families with young children, when the adult smokers become smoke-free, the benefits are felt by the entire household, both in terms of health improvement and the economic relief of no longer needing expensive medical treatments.

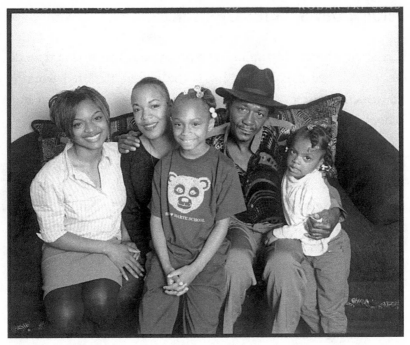

Marsha Akins and Jerome Davis with family

Photo by Kallsen and Harding

Jerome Davis, in His Own Voice

Texas is my home. My mom was a private-duty nurse. Hard work. Very hard. Seven kids, but I was the oldest. I started working construction [after school] when I was fourteen. And then I quit school when I was seventeen.

Mom had cancer in her stomach. She used to smoke. Smoked for quite a while; she stopped when she was about thirty-five. We probably could have had her longer if she didn't smoke cigarettes.

I was eighteen when I started smoking. I was from the city and my uncle stayed in the country. He asked me did I smoke. He said: "You ought to try a cigarette. After you get through eating, it makes you just relax." So he talked me into it, and then I smoked a cigarette and then the next day I smoked some more. And then it just got so I had the habit and just was smoking.

During that time—that was back in 1961–1962—we didn't have too much information about cigarettes and cancer. I got hooked right away. Maybe about a week, and I started buying me a pack. After time went on, I started smoking a pack and a half a day. And it went on like that until I went up to two packs a day. I had started drinking, too. And when you drink, you smoke more cigarettes; you just keep burning them up.

My mother didn't know I was smoking. I didn't want her to know. But when I got to be about nineteen, I started smoking in front of her. And she told me, "Cigarettes are not good for you; I don't want you smoking."

I started smoking Winstons. I switched to Kools. It was a better taste. It feels refreshing to your throat. I didn't have the money all the time to buy Kool cigarettes and sometimes I'd buy the one that you have to roll, Bugle. And sometimes I didn't have money for Bugles. I used to pick them up off the ground. Pick off the part that been in people's mouths. I used to go around to the ashtrays in public places and get me a bag and pick me up some butts and buy me some cigarette papers and roll up something and smoke. I was hooked. I didn't have the money all the time, but I would still smoke. Whole lot of times, [I] used to do without eating, and buy cigarettes.

I couldn't stop. Cigarettes are just like drugs: you get on them and you need help to stop. Down through the years, I started losing my relatives through smoking cigarettes, but I just kept on smoking. I lost my mother, I lost my brother, Uncle Junior, and then my Auntie Anell—she died with cancer, and she used to smoke. And my Uncle Bennie, he died with throat cancer. My mother, she died from cancer, and also my father. I know cigarettes are dangerous and no good for you. I know they will kill you, shorten your life if you continue to smoke. I've got proof. My relatives are gone from cigarettes, and so that is why I wanted to stop smoking. Cigarettes were killing my folks, all the people I love.

I cut down a bit, but I couldn't stop. I told my doctor I wanted to stop, so she told me about the smoking programs, and she signed me up. I made my mind up to put the patches on me. I craved for cigarettes, but I didn't smoke. It has been a year and a half since I had a cigarette.

Sometimes I still have an urge to pick it up, to smoke, but I just let it bypass. I don't smoke. Like I tell Marsha, she says, "Jerome, I dreamed that I was gonna smoke a cigarette," and I say, "Marsha, just blow that dream out of your mind cause it's not gonna do you no good. We gonna stick to our program, we are not gonna smoke." It has been working. She has been support for me, and I have been support for her. It makes me feel good that I don't have to pick them up.

I used to drink alcohol to solve my problems. It don't solve anything. I made my mind up when Marsha got the baby taken, and she needed my support. I said, "Marsha, what I am going to do is I am going to stop drinking. I am going to be your support." That is when I stopped. I had a reason to stop, so I stopped.

" I had a reason to stop, so I stopped. "

My only problem has been alcohol and cigarettes. I used to get locked up and go to jail, sometimes 45 days, without a cigarette. You would think 45 days, you would kick the habit, but your mind is not made up to stop smoking. So I get out of jail, and I have money and buy me two packs of cigarettes, and in about three hours, I have smoked them up. I had to get that nicotine back in.

I heard on the news that the doctor said cigarettes will give you cancer. I wanted to stop. I tried to stop smoking about two or three years after I started. But there wasn't no help out there for me. I listened to the radio; they said, "Today is the day for a smoke-out; go one day without smoking cigarettes." For ten years, I tried to do that. I couldn't do it. I would go a couple of hours and I couldn't. I wanted to, but I couldn't. I just take one day at a time, and that is the way I been doing it. You've got to be careful all the time. If I smoke me a cigarette right now, I have to start smoking again and start buying them. With coffee and with food and with driving around in my truck. I do have a desire to smoke, sometimes. I say, "No, I ain't gonna smoke no more," and it just go away.

Another reason why I don't: I want Marsha to stop. I help Marsha and Marsha helps me. Every morning I wake, and where I used to be tired, now I can get up and just go. I feel good. I breathe better. That is the truth. And when people come into our house, I tell them straight out, "You know you can't smoke in here; you have to go outside."

I come from a real, real big family. My family, when I was growing up, we all stuck together. I have raised my brothers and sisters. This is how I know about kids. I have been a kid, and I been hurt down the years, and my mommy and daddy separated, and I didn't want to see that. Marsha's oldest daughter, she came to me one time. She said, "Jerome, I want to thank you for getting my family, our family, back together, my mom." That is something for a seventeen-year-old to tell you that makes you feel really good.

It is a manmade thing why we are dying because of cigarette

smoke. My grandfather smoked, my father smoked, my mother smoked, my uncle smoked, and they all died from cancer. I wanted to stop because I said that cigarettes are not good for you, and they are killing all my people. Cigarettes will kill you. If you smoke cigarettes and keep on smoking cigarettes, they are gonna kill you. Cigarettes ain't no joke: they take you away before your time.

Who besides Jerome was affected by his smoking?

Jerome was a powerful healing force for his family. By taking care of himself and quitting smoking, he became a role model for his wife and improved the quality of health and life for his whole family.

Marsha Akins, in Her Own Voice

I've been through drugs, crack cocaine. Cigarette smoking is the worst habit I ever had. When I stopped crack cocaine, I was on my own, pregnant, and tired of being homeless. I was a lonely person, something waiting just to be knocked off the cliff.

I got started on the drugs with my daughter's father. I was eighteen, and he was twenty-eight. From then on, all the way up until I was twenty-nine, it was a life of drugs. I went into a program and stayed clean for three and a half years and then I relapsed. I was two months pregnant with Markala. I relapsed and met Jerome. We hit it off, me and Jerome. He was somebody that I could talk to.

Until Jerome, most of the people that I knew who stopped smoking just stopped. He said, "I went to smoking class today." I didn't want to hear that. "Oh no, I won't have a smoking partner anymore." That was my feeling, because Jerome and I did everything together. We agree on a lot of things, but this was going to be one thing that I wasn't going to agree on, because I wasn't ready for it. But here he was, putting reality on my mind, and it was something that I did not want to face. He said, "I don't want to die early; I want to live a long time and smoking is going to contribute to shortening my life. So I been going to this class, and I am going to get the patch, and I am going to stop smoking." I was scared 'cause all through my life, everybody I was around was smoking. But now I am hearing somebody that I am living in the same house with telling me that they no longer want to smoke.

As time went on, Jerome started doing the little steps before you stop smoking, and it was bothering me because I was saying to myself, "What is going to happen when he stops?" He didn't pressure me, he didn't argue, he didn't act different, he was the same Jerome. He was always positive. He wanted to stop smoking, and he started with step one. He didn't complain, but he was honest. I would say, "Jerome, you ever want a cigarette?" and he would say, "Yeah, Marsha, all the time, but I know that I have this patch on, and I know that I can't have a cigarette." He had made up his mind; he was finished smoking. I saw him going through these steps, and I didn't see him pulling his hair out. I didn't think it was possible to quit smoking without going through a lot of stress, and he didn't seem stressed out. So, I just kept it in my mind: "If he can do it, I can do it." I had to have somebody to follow, and he was somebody to follow.

My children have asthma. I know that to smoke around them is contributing to making it worse, but I couldn't stop. That was hurting me more than anything. Markala is three, Malane is seven, and Manesha is eighteen years old. Markala would get the asthma treatments. When I had to give her the treatments, I was miserable— giving her a treatment, and smoking. I'd get the machine out, plug it all up, fix the medication, and have her just sit there and be quiet. And I would run out and smoke a cigarette. That was terrible, really terrible.

> "I was more in fear of what I would go through than what would happen if I did smoke. Something was about to be taken from me that I had been doing all of my life."

When Jerome stopped smoking, I found myself very uncomfortable in this house. I didn't want to smoke in front of him. I was afraid to put the patch on, because I still wanted to smoke. Jerome had said once you put the patch on, you're not supposed to smoke. I was more in fear of what I would go through than what would happen if I did smoke. Something was about to be taken from me that I had been doing all of my life. What was I about to go through without it? I didn't know what I was heading for. All I knew was that if I did stop smoking, it would be better for my children's health; it would kind of eliminate the chances of me getting cancer.

My brother passed from cancer at the age of forty-four. My mother passed at the age of fifty-four. She smoked back-to-back. You could see it all over her face that she really wished she could put those cigarettes down. Before I got hooked on cigarettes, I would think: "Why don't you just stop; just put them down?" When I started smoking at thirteen, I was hooked so fast I could not believe it. I thought any time I wanted to, I could put the cigarettes down, but that is not the way it was. As a result of not wanting to believe I was hooked, when people would ask me, "Why do you smoke?" I would say, "Because I just want to." I never admitted that I didn't think that I could stop. I don't remember ever going two days without a cigarette.

When I had my hand going back and forth and blowing the smoke out of my mouth, I could act like things were not bothering me. I put my thought into the cigarette. I had my hand busy, and that taste from the cigarette was enough there for a minute to take me away from whatever, and then the cigarette was gone, and the problem was there.

A cigarette would interrupt whatever I was doing. If it was homework, I would start my homework, but I would stop to go light that cigarette, so I wasn't really concentrating on things I was doing. Most of the time when people were talking to me, I was thinking about a cigarette. I wasn't hearing half of what they were telling me.

When I would walk out the front door, I would light a cigarette as soon as I hit the bottom of the stairs, and I would walk to the bus stop with that cigarette. If the bus wasn't coming, I would light another one. I believed I would suffer to no end without smoking. I could not imagine living without smoking cigarettes, so I could not do it for me. I had to do it for somebody that I could see that I was harming. I didn't see myself harming myself unless cancer would have shown up. That would have been the only thing that would have alerted me that smoking is bad for your health. But listening to my daughter, listening to my baby wheeze, I felt guilty.

I was uncomfortable all of my life smoking a cigarette. When I would come home after getting off the bus, walking down the street with a cigarette, I'd find it hard to look for my key to open the door. I had to smoke the cigarette first and then I would be angry with myself because I didn't enjoy that cigarette, so now when I get into the house, I have to light another. Walking out the house carrying Markala, if Jerome was walking with me, I would have to ask him to hold Markala so that I could light a cigarette, and if he wanted to give her back to me, I would get mad because I didn't enjoy that cigarette, and I had to throw half of my cigarette away so I could take Markala back into my arms.

Everybody started getting on my case. Venisha would say, "Mommy, when you smoke cigarettes, I am getting second-hand smoke. So, would that mean that you don't care?" Jerome said, "Marsh, you ought to go outside when you are smoking." I didn't like having to leave the room and be in another room by myself. I got to the point that there was too much missing for me. My thought was, "I can't wait to get that patch." I put it on, and I gave myself an excuse to smoke again. So I took the patch off and started smoking. Next time, I made a date. I said, "I am going to put the patch on, follow the rules, and I am going to consider myself a person who is not smoking anymore. I am going to follow the steps." It would have been very easy to take the patch off and just go smoke a cigarette every time I had a problem. But I made a rule for myself: "I am going to give myself four days." I needed to remove everything out of the house, the ashtrays, cigarettes, the old cigarette packs in my purses, everything.

After the second day, I was shocked cause I was able to say, "I haven't had a cigarette for two days, which tells me that I am smoke-free. I don't have the urge that I thought I was going to have, and I guess it is the patch that is helping." But all the things that I thought were going to happen, like the world crashing down on me, did not happen.

During the time I was smoking, I could never picture telling my children that smoking is bad for your health, 'cause I was doing it. How can you tell a child not to pick up a cigarette when here you are, smoking? You put a cigarette before them: "Wait a minute, I have to go have a cigarette; leave me alone, I've got to go smoke my cigarette." Now I do not put that cigarette before my children; therefore, I can be their role model. I feel really good Markala has not had an asthma attack, has not even wheezed in months. The smoke in the house was the big factor contributing to her asthma and wheezing. She is getting better, not worse.

> "It is much harder to live with smoking than it is to live without smoking."

I am going to school for nursing. I don't think I would be able to do it if I was smoking cigarettes. The estimating and averaging-up things and putting things together with my hands that are important, and saving someone's life: I would probably be thinking about a cigarette at the same time. You have to be aware; your mind has to be open; you have to have your hands free. If I am thinking about a cigarette, I would not be able to do any of those things. I am really glad that I am not smoking, 'cause I get to be a nurse to the best of my ability. I am free to think about what it is I am doing. I can concentrate on the work I am doing. If I have a problem, I face the problem, I go all the way through it; I am not going to cut it off halfway and then go have a cigarette. I have time for myself. I have time to do so many things. I am more relaxed. I feel mature. I can express myself better. I get out of the house on time, I get to school on time; my cigarette is not holding me back. I don't have that "worry" feeling all the time.

When you put the cigarette down, your hands come alive, and they have all these things they want to do that the cigarettes were stopping them from doing. My hands were in prison; now they are free. Everything I did with that cigarette caused me to be uncomfortable, and all the time I was thinking I was being comfortable. It is much harder to live with smoking than it is to live without smoking.

Who besides Marsha Akins was affected by her smoking?

Marsha had a lot of courage, and even though she was afraid to quit smoking, she did it. With her newfound strength, she took better care of her family and even went back to school to earn a professional license. You can see in the stories and courage that Marsha and Jerome have shown how the action of one person can have a huge impact on the lives of many other people for years to come. This highlights the idea behind "social contagion": positive or negative behaviors can have a viral quality and affect networks of people. The change that Jerome and Marsha made could truly affect the health of their family and friends for generations, and this all started with the action of one person.

Who besides you is affected by your smoking?

Action steps for people who want to be smoke-free

Today, children are exposed to a great deal of information about tobacco and come home from school begging their parents to please stop smoking. It is a very uncomfortable feeling to be confronted by one's young children for doing something as indefensible as smoking. Many smokers are accustomed to medicating uncomfortable feelings with cigarettes, so it's not unusual for your children's pleas to trigger an urge to smoke. If you are caught in this loop, how could you respond most productively to the uncomfortable feelings you are experiencing? Rather than spiral into self-blame and hiding, seeking help to find a way out of your dilemma will liberate not only you but also the people who care about you.

In addition to caring about yourself, sometimes it helps to think about how smoking impacts the people in your life. Protecting them could also help you protect yourself. What kind of a role model do you want to be for the young people in your life? Second-hand smoke is a recognized danger, even more so for young children; thinking of protecting them could also help you to protect yourself.

> "Rather than spiral into self-blame and hiding, seeking help to find a way out of your dilemma will liberate not only you but also the people who care about you."

Who are the people (or pets) in your life who stand to be most affected by your smoking? There may be some people whose health is put at risk because of exposure to second- and third-hand smoke. There may also be people who will be impacted if you become ill from smoking, and they are faced with the burden of caring for you. Even worse, they may grieve losing you to a smoking-related disease. Smoking is a social problem that impacts more than the smoker. Thinking about this aspect of the disease might make you feel very uncomfortable, so perhaps you block these thoughts and feelings. You may even cope with the discomfort by smoking.

There is another way to cope: Look at what steps you might take toward real smoke-free comfort (as opposed to the false comfort in cigarettes). **It's much easier to live without the fear and the worry that comes with smoking.** If you feel overwhelmed by the challenge of stopping smoking, start with simple steps. If you smoke in your home, find a place to smoke outside and smoke only there. If you smoke in your car, cut drinking straws to the length of a cigarette to take with you when you drive, and do deep breathing instead. Change your brand of cigarette and cut down by one or two every day. Even small changes will give you a sense of accomplishment. As you continue to limit where and when you smoke, you will move forward to a time when you will no longer be burdened by the demands and disturbance of living with tobacco dependence.

Three Key Points

1. Smoking is never just about one person; it affects anyone who is exposed to it or who cares about what is happening to the smoker.

2. Quitting smoking may be the lightning rod of motivation to inspire someone near and dear to you to do the same.

3. Children (and pets) of smokers suffer more health problems and missed school than those of nonsmokers. As a nonsmoker, you can raise a better-educated, healthier, and happier child.

NOTES

CHAPTER SEVEN

What is your power and how do you choose to use it?

Think about it: don't you often start smoking as a quick way to get something that might otherwise seem out of your reach? For example, some people start smoking because they identify with a role model they want to be like. Andy Ficaro, one of the subjects in this chapter, started smoking by lighting his father's cigarette butts because, like many sons, he wanted to be like his father. Some people smoke to become a member of a peer group, either real (friends) or imagined (movie stars). Others, like Jenny Bender, start smoking to give voice to social or personal dissatisfaction or disenchantment. Without being aware of the freedoms you are losing by involving yourself with cigarettes, you naively get entrapped with something that can hold you captive for decades.

When smokers become more familiar with the nature of the tobacco industry, many are horrified about where their money is going. The industry is built on tricks and lies. For years, tobacco companies covered up the true effects of smoking (addiction and disease) so that they could continue to make enormous profits at the expense of their consumers' health. Cigarette manufacturing is an industry without regard for its consumers' well-being, an industry that capitalizes on our insecurities and various class and racial inequalities. For example, advertisements show smokers who are enjoying competitive sports, when, in fact, smoking limits your ability to participate in rigorous exercise. Smoking is often equated with being sexy and free, when the residue of smoking on clothing and breath is the opposite of sexiness and many smokers testify to feeling trapped by smoking.

By smoking, you give away your real power in exchange for a fantasy. What powers are you looking for in your decision to smoke? What powers do you lose?

If you consider that money is power, how could you choose to use your power in a way that is a more accurate expression of your values? Perhaps you want to buy some music so that you can dance around your house with abandon. Or you might want to sign up for a class to learn something creative or save for a trip to someplace you've long wanted to visit.

We have to continually be jumping off cliffs
and developing our wings on the way down.
Kurt Vonnegut

Andy Ficaro

Andy had an abundance of wealth and resources to use in his effort to cope with lung cancer. A successful, self-made businessman in the software industry, Andy cut a dapper figure in his finely tailored Italian suits and expensive shoes. Impeccably groomed, he had the air of a man of means and power. And yet, he was powerless over his fate and paid a heavy price for his smoking. He turned his sense of powerlessness against what he saw as the root of the evil that had overtaken him: the tobacco industry. When smokers learn more about the companies that produce cigarettes and manipulate young people into experimenting with smoking, their outrage can be a source of energy to stop smoking. More than 430,000 Americans die every year from smoking-related diseases; that's the equivalent of three jumbo jets crashing every day of the year. If an airline company crashed a single jet every day for a week—much less a year—it's unlikely that passengers would continue to climb on board. And yet, the tobacco companies continue to successfully peddle their deadly products.

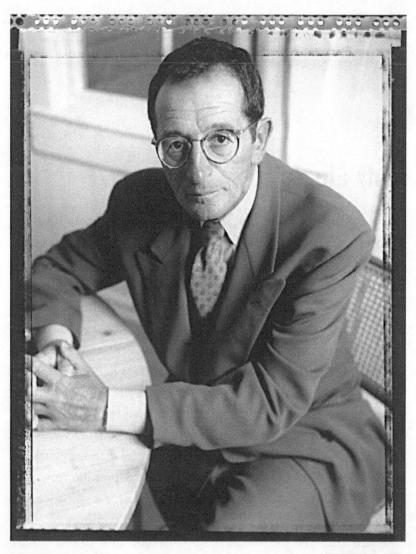

Andrew Ficaro   Photo by John Harding

Andrew Ficaro, in His Own Voice

I am 58 years old, Italian, born on the South Side of Chicago. My mother was a housewife. My father, by trade, was a theater projectionist and would also work at either a restaurant or a liquor store or apartment buildings or some combination of those three things. I graduated from law school. I have a small software company, and we design and sell routing software.

I began smoking at the nice age of four. I used to take my father's butts out of the ashtray, go in the bathroom, and smoke them. I started buying cigarettes by the age of six. I would hide them outside at night and then, on my way to school in the morning, I would smoke my first cigarette. When it rained, that was kind of a bummer because then my cigarettes got wet. By the time I was nine years old, there were a lot of kids in the neighborhood [who] smoked. It was easy to buy cigarettes. You just went to the corner grocery store and bought them. The grocer just assumed it was for your parents.

When I was 35 years old, I did manage to quit smoking for a year. I was making so much money so fast that it dawned on me: "What in the world am I going to do if I get sick and die from smoking these cigarettes? I won't be able to spend this money fast enough. I won't be able to enjoy it." I quit by weaning myself on to cigars. I was doing a lot of travel in Canada at the time and was able to buy the Cuban cigars.

I smoked cigars for a month and then every two or three weeks. I was able to quit cigarettes for a year and I felt terrific. I woke up in the morning instantly alert no matter how much I had drunk the night before. Then, when I was playing poker, I reached out and grabbed one, and that was it. Within a couple of days, I went right back up to two packs a day. In the morning as soon as

I woke up, the only thing that would stop me from coughing was a cigarette.

I tried to quit numerous times by reducing. I would say: "OK, I am only going to smoke a cigarette every half hour." And I would do that for two days and then say, "OK, now I am only going to smoke every forty-five minutes and now I am only going to smoke every hour," and I would bullshit myself until I would get down to anywhere from four to eight cigarettes a day, which is terrific coming from forty. But something would happen, and I would just go right back up again.

The middle of November, I went in for a physical. My doctor told me to come in every year since I was a smoker, but I would come in every two or three years. This one was every three years. A physical, routine chest x-ray and that is when he found the tumor. I had no symptoms.

I have gone through five radiation treatments so far. I refused chemotherapy under any circumstance. They have done the brain scan and the bone scans and the CT scans; and according to all those scans, other than one supposedly tiny, tiny bit of cancer in the lymph nodes, the cancer has not spread.

The radiation can shrink the size of the tumor. The chemotherapy acts as an insurance policy. Chemotherapy doesn't buy me that much versus the downside of it. If my odds of survival are 20 to 30 percent to beat this, and the chemotherapy isn't adding that much to it in combination with radiation, what is the point?

You have to want to, and even after I was diagnosed with lung cancer, I couldn't quit. I mean I *couldn't* quit. My best friend would just constantly tell me, "You have to want to do it."

I tried to reduce smoking. I was disappointed that I couldn't quit. You say to yourself, "What difference does it make?" You go up and down. "I have cancer, I am going to die, so what is the point in not smoking or smoking?" You adopt different attitudes at different points in time.

I left for Hawaii. I took sixteen packs of cigarettes with me and I also took the Nicotrol inhaler. Before I went to bed, I didn't have any conscious thought that this was going to be my last cigarette. I woke up the next morning, tried the Nicotrol inhaler and it helped. It gives you a little bit of the same rush that the cigarette does. You are holding it in between your fingers so it feels like a cigarette and it looks like a cigarette, you are dragging on it. I could feel the nicotine going in, I could feel it and it certainly eliminates the toughest portion, the physical addictiveness.

I ran into a guy in Hawaii who was a world-class poker player from Alaska. World class. He told me one of the tricks to use is your imagination. Just imagine that you are not a smoker anymore. When that urge is really strong and you want that cigarette, you have to think about the fact that you are going to repeat everything you did before and start quitting smoking all over again.

> "I was doing something that was obviously terrible to myself and I didn't enjoy it."

My best friend told me, "It ain't the caboose that kills you," it's that first cigarette. So I would fight the urge and I wouldn't have it.

I strongly recommend the Nicotrol inhaler. The first day was kind of easy because it was so novel. Days two, three, four, and five were awfully, awfully tough. There are still certain points during the day, it's a bitch. I want a cigarette so bad sometimes I want to rip my head off. That is not pleasant.

The ugly part of it was, I never enjoyed smoking. Maybe a long, long time ago I did, but I didn't like the taste of it, I didn't like what it was doing to me, it didn't make me feel good. So I was doing something that was obviously terrible to myself and I didn't enjoy it.

Up until three, four, or five years ago, I did not believe that tobacco was physically addictive. I believed it was strictly a mental addiction and I just was one of those people who couldn't quit. Cocaine was easy to quit. I smoked marijuana every single day since I was probably 25 years old, and five or six years ago, I stopped. I had no withdrawal and I was furious that I could stop smoking something I truly loved and couldn't stop smoking cigarettes, which I truly hated. I was furious with myself. In the early movies that you saw about heroin, the message came across loud and clear: you use it once and you are hooked for life; you are hooked forever. That made a difference in terms of deterring me. If I had gotten that kind of a message about nicotine, maybe that would have made a difference to me.

This government fining of the tobacco industries is the biggest sham that could be perpetrated on people that there is. You've got to just pull the business and be done with it. Everything else is bullshit; everything else is trying to fix the fix with a fix. I am a good example of somebody being diagnosed with lung cancer and told, "You are going to have a tough time with this operation if you don't quit smoking. Smoking will make recovery and healing much harder." I still couldn't quit smoking. Do you think that taxing the cigarettes an extra fifty fucking cents is going to make me stop smoking? You fine Tobacco Company X millions of dollars and they turn around and pass it back on to me. That is a sham. If you are going to fine them, then fine them with their own money, not with my money. I don't know what they fined the tobacco companies, but fine them a hundred times that amount and make them raise the price of cigarettes to twenty dollars a pack. That might have an effect.

The best way to get people to quit is put the companies out of business. If this is truly a life-threatening disease, if there can be no more argument that cigarettes kill people in the numbers they do, then just ban it. Be done with it.

What was Andy's power and how did he choose to use it?

Andy turned his outrage, anger, and despair about a cancer diagnosis against the core of the deadly tobacco epidemic: the cigarette industry. He recognized that even with increasing knowledge about the health effects of smoking, there would always be people who fall prey to industry tactics. To fuel his rejection of continued smoking, he used his outrage at being duped and used by an industry that kills one-third of its customers. He saw that his power had been robbed from him and he was determined to fight back.

It's not that I'm so smart. It's just that I stay with problems longer. **Albert Einstein**

Jenny Bender

Like many young people, Jenny was convinced that she could experiment with smoking and not get hooked; her sense of personal power in relation to cigarettes was distorted. Her beliefs proved to be unfounded when she experienced the harm that smoking can cause to someone with asthma and she kept on smoking.

Jenny used cigarettes to medicate anxiety and depression, so when she eventually tried to stop, those symptoms kept leading her back to smoking. The fact that most of her friends smoked made it harder to think about quitting. Weekend activities typically included going to bars to socialize and hang out and, at the time in Manhattan, the city where she lived, smoking was pervasive in most public places. What could she do to substitute for the activity that occupied her hands and managed her anxiety? Jenny decided to take up knitting and would tote her various projects with her; as her friends smoked and socialized, she knitted and enjoyed their company.

Jenny started smoking as a teenager partly as rebellion and partly to fit in with the outsider crowd she identified with. In some respects, smoking arrested her emotional development. Rather than grow to learn how to deal with negative feelings, she used cigarettes to blunt her discomfort. When she stopped smoking, she was pushed to learn skills to help alleviate anxiety and worked to make a contribution to change a world she found so dissatisfying.

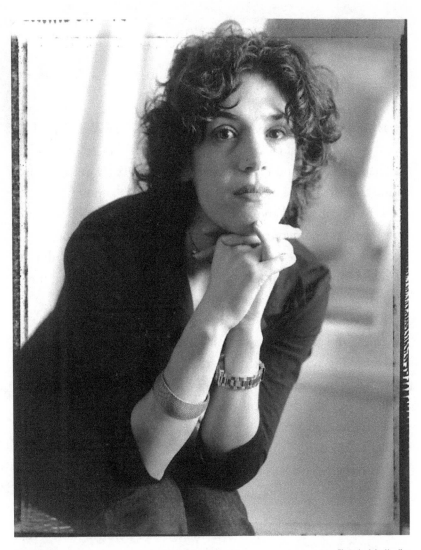

Jenny Bender

Photo by John Harding

Jenny Bender, in Her Own Voice

I was born and raised in San Francisco. I live in New York City. I am twenty-five. My first cigarette: I was thirteen and in eighth grade. I had had a bad day and I had a pack of my friend's cigarettes. I came home and tried smoking for the first time. I was alone.

I was depressed and angry at anyone who was in a position of power and was someone who I thought abused it. I was completely overcome by rage at injustice. Most of that anger got turned in on myself. There was no other place to put it, and it ate away at me. It tormented me. I was in agony.

I was rebelling against my parents, my teachers, against all the rules, and the feelings of not being able to take control of my life. Smoking was this exciting, risky, private thing. I got to feel powerful, and like I had this secret that was adventurous and just mine. It was like dessert all the time: have a great meal and then have a cigarette; watch a great movie, listen to a great song, and smoke a cigarette.

I remember not wanting to hear what my mother had to say and thinking that I didn't think that I would get hooked because I didn't feel hooked and because I knew that it wasn't smart. I wasn't in touch with myself, even though I thought that I was. I just didn't know what to do with too many feelings and thoughts. It was a lot easier to be somewhat tuned out.

"Tobacco is one way of having a sense of control: "I have my own life and you don't know about it; I am making my own decisions."

Tobacco is one way of having a sense of control: "I have my own life and you don't know about it; I am making my own decisions." Change this culture, and that will change that reality. If teenagers had more control, they wouldn't be so drawn to tobacco and other drugs.

I got hooked. The feeling of excitement and the feeling of intensity and of having a best friend and the feeling of things being twice as enjoyable—that was the addiction.

My mother was very supportive. I was not allowed to smoke in the house or anywhere the smoke would come near the house, but she knew that I smoked. It was clear she cared, that she didn't want me to smoke, but there wasn't judgment. She always said, "When you feel ready to quit, I want to help." It was never, "You really need to stop doing this; this is really bad for you," 'cause obviously anybody who smokes knows that. They know it is bad for you.

I struggled with cigarettes all through high school and college. It was always something I knew I wanted to stop. It was exciting, but it was never the lifestyle that I wanted; it was never who I wanted to be. I didn't want the addiction, I didn't want to be controlled by something outside of myself, and I didn't want to be out of my head and out of my body.

I said I would quit after college. I quit for a while and then I moved to New York. I would smoke when I went out, and then I was smoking all the time again. I would smoke for two months and quit for two months and then start up again. I needed to make a decision: either smoke or work on my asthma. What pushed me to quit once and for all was when I started to work on my health.

I can't believe I smoked for so long, with asthma. I would use my inhaler so that I could smoke a cigarette. My senior year in college, my boyfriend had to take me to the infirmary in the middle of the night 'cause I couldn't breathe. I spent the night there and got treated, and the next night I was smoking again.

I stopped smoking, I started eating better, and I started working out more, this whole series of things aimed towards making my life feel mine. The first few days of not smoking, I would get terribly cranky and on edge. That was not what was hard; it was the emotional stuff and the habit of doing.

I have a hard time with anxiety. Just sitting and talking would be very difficult for me, but if I could sit and talk and smoke, then I would channel the anxious energy into the movement of the hand and the mouth. Knitting helped. I brought my knitting everywhere—even to the bar because it was the only way I could sit around with my friends and not have a cigarette. I could sit and have something to do with my hands and talk; it wasn't like painting or writing, where you had to be focused on what you were doing. It was like smoking: you could knit and do it.

> "I brought my knitting everywhere—even to the bar because it was the only way I could sit around with my friends and not have a cigarette."

Every once in a while, I crave a cigarette when I am with friends who are smoking, but it passes very quickly now. I never indulge in it; I don't play: "Maybe I should have just one." Because of asthma, [when I go] out where everybody smokes, I always wake up the next morning and feel sore in my chest. I am very allergic to the smoke; I get irritated and sneezy; my eyes get itchy. God, I just can't believe that I used to actually do this to myself every day!

Quitting smoking is one thing of many along a path of changing my life. I didn't quit smoking and all of a sudden everything was different, but I changed a lot of things, trying to be more focused on taking care of myself. I used to get sad and stressed-out and smoke a cigarette; now I get sad and stressed out and do an art project or go to the gym. I was always trying to get to the place where I am now; being a smoker just wouldn't fit with who I am. It doesn't jive with trying to live from a more aware place. Now I am trying to take care of myself rather than punish myself, trying to go to the root of what is happening, trying to move out of it rather than staying in the black hole of "life sucks." Smoking was kind of a way of [saying] "Oh fuck it! It is my life and it is my business and it all sucks out there." Now I am trying to change that: "It is my life and let me make the best of it."

Being addicted to cigarettes, as soon as you cross that boundary, all the control is gone and then everything, the entire focus, changes. It is amazing to me the extent to which that is true. If I go out and I am hanging out with friends, it is all about hanging out with friends. With smoking, it is all about when you are going to have that cigarette, and it completely pulls you out of the moment, out of yourself.

The realization and actualization of being in control of myself and my life is incredibly freeing. I feel proud of myself when I am out, and people offer me cigarettes and I say, "I don't smoke." I love being able to say that. I feel free, I feel healthier, my asthma is better; I used to feel sick and tired all the time. A sore throat and asthma was my normal state of being. When I first started getting healthier and stopped getting these things, the first time I felt sick I thought, "This is how I used to feel every day, every night, every morning. This is how I felt, and that was the way that I lived." I am much more aware, emotionally and physically, and I am not making decisions 'cause of an addiction.

What was Jenny's power and how did she choose to use it?

Jenny was not unlike many young people who fall prey to an industry that cautions, "Smoking is a decision to be made by adults, not children." Wanting to exercise what she mistook as a means to power and control by smoking, she had to first become smoke-free to be able to truly tap in to and develop her creative powers.

What is your power and how do you choose to use it?

Action steps for people who want to be smoke-free

Andy's story is one of many where a person smokes long enough to contract a severe, smoking-related disease and then feels outraged at the industry that encourages and profits from tobacco use. What do you know about the industry you support with your cigarette dollars?

Many smokers start smoking as an act of rebellion. That youthful rebellious energy is normal and healthy; how could you use it now to rebel against an industry and a product that wants to control you and has the potential to ruin your life? If money is power, how, other than smoking, might you choose to invest that power? Calculate the amount of money you spend on smoking in a year; how else might you like to spend that sum? After stopping smoking, you may well feel connected to a power that was hidden behind cigarettes. Many smokers who stop smoking discover a feeling of *"If I can do this, I can do anything."* They go on to give expression to that sense of power in creative and exciting ways.

> **Calculate the amount of money you spend on smoking in a year; how else might you like to spend that sum?**

Jenny's story documents a process of addressing feelings of powerlessness by taking on a behavior—smoking—that carries a facade of power. Unfortunately, the promise of control with cigarettes turns out to be the reality of being controlled. In my own experience, one of the reasons I used cigarettes was to create boundaries in social situations. With a cigarette in my hand, I could artfully define the distance I needed between me and someone else to feel comfortable and safe. One of the things I had to learn as a nonsmoker was how to feel justified in setting and maintaining boundaries. Learning to do this was a process of reclaiming personal power.

> What are some of the ways in which you have used cigarettes to manage fears, insecurities, or powerlessness? Take a few moments to write down your thoughts on the chapter notes page.

Jenny eventually began to reverse her sense of powerlessness by becoming politically active. She joined with other students at her college to fight for the rights of welfare mothers, and, in the years since, she has channeled that former sense of powerlessness into standing up for whom she cares about and what she believes in.

What are some of the ways in which you have used cigarettes to manage fears, insecurities, or powerlessness? Take a few moments to write down your thoughts here. Once you have a list, begin to explore some of your options for addressing these vulnerable feelings without cigarettes. Some of us who are shy and have used cigarettes to boost self-confidence have joined groups like Toastmasters International to practice feeling more at ease in public situations. Others have found groups to join where people shared interests, like hiking or other sports.

There is an exercise we teach in the stop-smoking program to help participants get in touch with personal courage. People are invited to remember an experience when there was something they wanted to do in spite of doubts about their ability to do it. They get in touch with the inner resources they then tapped into to accomplish their courageous act. In spite of their doubts or fears, they made those goals happen.

Quitting smoking takes courage! At different times in our lives, we have all shown courage and have been inspired by the courage of others. It can be helpful to remember these times and use them as you begin the quitting process. Take some time to reflect and record your thoughts.

Courage = Desire + Doubt + Action

There is an exhilaration that comes in facing head-on the hard truths and saying, "I will not give up. It may take a long time, but I will find a way to prevail." Jim Collins, Good to Great

To do something about which you have little confidence requires courage. While you're smoking, you often stop short of stretching your limits or testing yourself. **What are some things you would think about doing if you stepped outside your comfort zone?** Without being aware of it, this is another place where you might have been using cigarettes to hold yourself back.

Three Key Points

1. Smoking can keep you from experiencing your authentic personal power.

2. The tobacco industry exploits a sense of powerlessness and encourages smoking as a way to compensate.

3. Stopping smoking opens the possibility of feeling truly powerful: "If I can stop smoking, I can do anything."

My Courage Experiences	How I Can Use Them to Help Me Become Smoke-Free

NOTES

CHAPTER EIGHT

Who would you be without cigarettes?

Smokers can be intense people who use tobacco to keep powerful feelings under control. By relying on cigarettes to manage their emotions, they become less true to themselves and, over time, fall short of what they could become. Most smokers know that they use cigarettes to subdue negative emotions such as anger or stress. However, almost any emotion, positive or negative, can be a lot to handle, and the smoker typically relies on cigarettes to turn down the volume. When I was a smoker, if I was praised for something that I had done well, the feelings of reward were sometimes stronger than what I could handle, so I would light a cigarette to bring good feelings to a tolerable level. Feeling "too good" can be threatening, and a cigarette can control that threat.

All of the individuals in this chapter are impressive for the vivid spectrum of their strong personalities. And as all of them moved toward becoming non-smokers, qualities emerged and blossomed, changing how they experience and live their lives.

Be aware of your breathing. Notice how this takes attention away from your thinking and creates space. **Eckhart Tolle**

Barbara Vos

Barbara Vos has a powerful ability to focus, analyze, and create. She is a successful painter, she is a superb cook, and she makes an art of friendship. Barbara joined the program with two friends, one of whom would eventually become her husband. She was one of the few who regularly practiced every single tool that was offered to her over an eight-week counseling period, and she emerged with a system she used for years. Although she was drawn to becoming smoke-free for a number of reasons, it was her asthma that finally drove her to learn to quit.

When I first met Barbara, she was attending tai chi classes several times a week. She also started swimming as part of her preparation to stop smoking. As she cut down on smoking and eventually stopped, she found that exercise helped her to improve her breathing capacity and boosted her mood. Of course, that advance was made easier by the fact that it was impossible to smoke and swim at the same time. Swimming also increased her awareness of the quality of her breathing. When she was a smoker, engaging in activities that called attention to how smoking harmed her ability to breathe deeply made her anxious, so she avoided exertion.

Barbara's rich emotional life had been held in check with smoking. When she first stopped, she was overwhelmed with confusion. How could she paint without a cigarette in her hand? How could she think and create without whirls of smoke in the air around her? Powerful feelings threatened to drag her down. But instead of returning to cigarettes to help her cope, she responded by increasing her exercise and pushing herself to express her feelings in Group. Even though she felt uncomfortable without cigarettes, she refused to be deterred from her goal and steadfastly persevered. It was a joy to witness her physical health improve, and even more to observe the growing depth of her self-acceptance. By nature, Barbara is drawn to self-exploration; without the distancing effects of tobacco, her relationship with herself only became deeper.

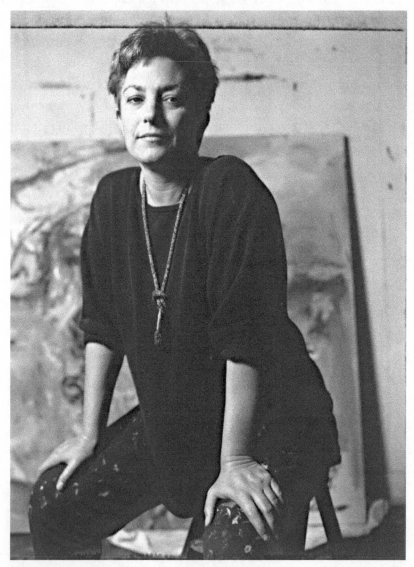

Barbara Vos

Photo by John Harding

Barbara Vos, in Her Own Voice

I was born in Long Island, New York, but I grew up in Brooklyn. I've lived in San Francisco since 1976, the year after my mother died. When my mother found out that she had reticulum cell sarcoma, a rare form of cancer, I returned home to take care of her. The cancer killed her in six months. She was a smoker, and she never quit. I always felt that smoking contributed to her death. A pack and a half, two packs a day—that was how she smoked. She was in a cloud all the time. I was breathing secondhand smoke my whole life. I hated my mother's smoking, so, of course, I thought I'd never smoke.

When I was in art school, I started rolling cigarettes for a friend. I'm very dexterous, and I like doing things with my hands. It was winter. I smoked just one cigarette that was rolled, and I felt tough, tomboyish. On my own, at age seventeen, in college, I was scared. Smoking definitely has a lot to do with maintaining a stance to stave off fear. You leave home for college and two months later, you're smoking, the first time you're away from the person who smokes a lot.

I hold a lot of anxieties in my upper respiratory system and my shoulders. Whenever I focused on my breath, I would have anxiety because of all the years of smoking, but also because I had asthma. I remember having an asthma attack and my mother next to me, smoking. I remember walking in the country in some pristine, beautiful place and the fog, the mist in the morning, so frail and fragrant, and being engulfed by the smell of cigarette smoke. I remember feeling depressed to have her trailing behind everybody to hide that she was smoking. My mother had a lot of shame, and she added smoking into her big lot of shame . If you too already have shame in you, smoking comes in pretty handy. It isn't a way of truly dealing with the shame, but it is a way of letting that pain be there and suffering with it.

She always wanted to quit. She never could, and as part of that pattern of wanting to quit and not being able to, I felt like I was her. I was doing the same thing she did. I was keeping her alive by smoking. What made it so hard for me to quit was letting go of her and of doing something that she hadn't. I couldn't let go of that.

What changed for me was having a steady, stable place with all kinds of people with different stories—a place where people were trying to be truthful and open and were trying to get help to do something that they needed and wanted to do. It is what got me to quit: going through all of the practice, doing all of the exercises, and really letting stopping smoking be the focus. You have to focus on not smoking and do good things for yourself that help you not smoke. When you're troubled, it's hard to do good things for yourself instead of smoking, so you must start from a positive place. That means taking care of yourself, which was hard for me to do.

Before, I used to say, "Oh well, I think I'll exercise," and then I'd go have a cigarette. You can't exercise right after you have a cigarette. I never did aerobic exercise until about three months ago, nor did I know what it was really like to sweat. Deep abdominal breathing is too scary if you are a smoker. You just can't do it because when you're taking an abdominal breath, you're thinking about your body. I have a chance now to have another body, to have a healthy body. My breathing has changed a lot. I can relax. My diaphragm used to hurt all the time; now I can relax it. I feel a spaciousness in my lungs. That is just one of the best things about quitting smoking. Only now am I beginning to know what it really feels like to be relaxed. Smoking is the fool's relaxation.

> "Only now am I beginning to know what it really feels like to be relaxed. Smoking is the fool's relaxation."

There's so much pain in smoking. In fact, it reminds you of your pain. If a terrible thing happens, a crisis, and you start smoking, it just keeps reminding you of that crisis. I used to think there was something wrong about being in a bad mood and that I should have a cigarette. Now I still get in bad moods and I still don't like it, but I'm also more willing not to be perfect. More important, I don't think about smoking a cigarette because of my disappointment at not being perfect. I feel much freer from that repetition of anxiety and pain.

As a non-smoker, you can focus and be in something longer, so it pushes your limits a little more. Your anxiety might come but then it lessens, and you're still staying with it. You are also able to develop more feelings, like feeling lonely. Things that would be controlled by lighting a cigarette can, instead, be explored and then solved in some way. To realize that you're mad at somebody and to let that feeling be fluid, not keep it at a distance, not decide "okay, well, I'm mad" and just puff away at a cigarette: that's a victory.

That's an amazing thing: to let the natural course of an emotion go free, without trying to control it with cigarettes.

Who would Barbara be without cigarettes?

Barbara used tobacco to keep powerful feelings under control, beginning in college when she first started smoking to stave off the fear of being on her own for the first time. And, like her mother, Barbara's cigarettes provided her an easy magnet for any shameful feelings. As long as she was a smoker, she had something to be ashamed of and that shame was an anchor for other shameful feelings. She even used smoking to help cope with the anxiety she felt as a result of smoking-related health concerns.

When Barbara quit smoking, who she was and how she lived changed: she became someone who exercises. She learned how to truly relax. She also learned how to sit with and express uncomfortable feelings instead of trying to cover them up.

Find the seed
at the bottom of your heart
and bring forth
a flower
Shigenori Kameoka

Clarence Brown

In 1984, when I first began working as a primary care nurse in the San Francisco General Hospital Adult Outpatient Medical Clinic, Clarence Brown was one of my most challenging patients. Already stricken with multiple and complex medical problems, Clarence was nearly impossible to manage, and he persistently tried my patience and stretched the limits of my compassion. Because several of his problems affected his breathing, it was important that he show up for his regular follow-up appointments to try to get his symptoms under control. But he would invariably miss his scheduled appointment and then show up at the clinic near closing time, gasping for breath and demanding treatment. In addition to being medically difficult, he was grumpy, rude, and dismissive of my attempts to engage him in staying alive.

A heavy smoker, Clarence had been on life support eight times by 1989. In his own words, he was a cat who had used up eight of his nine lives. In 1990, he made up his mind to "get off the fast-moving train headed for a steep cliff and take a ride on a slow-moving turtle." He decided to stop smoking. By March 1991, he was smoke-free.

Over time, Clarence became the beloved patriarch of the smoking-cessation program, saving lives by telling his story and inspiring other smokers to quit smoking. Clarence's testimony proved that there is no such thing as a hopeless case when it comes to becoming smoke-free and turning your life around. With his charismatic personality and generous spirit, it was easy for him to make good on a promise he had made to himself that he would make at least three people smile every day. Larger than life, Clarence did everything grandly.

More than a decade after he stopped smoking and about four months before he died, Clarence returned to being short-tempered and crabby. Over the years, he had become more responsive to my efforts to manage his care, coming to appointments on time and returning my calls when I would check up on how he was doing. But now, three or four messages would pile up before he called me back, and when he did show up at the clinic, he was irritable and impatient. During his smoke-free years, his mood was usually upbeat, regardless of how he felt physically, so the changes in his behavior were noteworthy. I worried that something was up.

One day, I asked: had he thought about smoking or had any smokes? After nearly eleven years of being a non-smoker, Clarence admitted he had been so upset about something happening in his family that he'd lashed out at someone, "Give me a smoke!" and his command had been obeyed. When he assured me this would not happen again, I was not convinced. I felt real concern, knowing how dangerous smoking could be to his survival.

Over the following weeks, other interactions confirmed my suspicions that tobacco was taking hold again in Clarence's life. When he lamented, "I know I've let you down, and I am sorry," I knew he was in trouble.

It took a while before he was willing to open up in the weekly Support Group. Here, Clarence was a legend. For so many years, he had shared his story and inspired smokers to stop killing themselves by smoking. He was our wise elder, our Rock of Gibraltar. One evening in Group, I looked across the room at him and said, "Do you want to work tonight?" He knew what I was asking and paused to consider before answering, "Okay, I'll do that."

"Are you smoking, Clarence?" I inquired.

"Yes."

"How often, and how much?"

"Over the weekend, I smoked a pack and a half."

Disturbance bubbled up as I watched a room full of men and women go into fear and denial.

"What?! What did he say?"

"You're joking, right?"

"How *could* you?"

Fear turned into anger as everyone scrambled to find safety from the danger they began to suspect had ensnared our hero. Clarence, shaken and confused, then acknowledged, "I'm smoking. It's terrible. Watch out, it can happen to anybody."

Our eyes met and locked as I heard myself say, "Clarence, you know that there is no one for whom I have more respect than you. And now you have done what I would not have thought possible: You have deepened that respect, made it greater. For here you are, giving us the last piece in this work. You are showing us how to come back to people for whom you are a leader and say 'I need help.' Could there be any greater strength or wisdom than this?"

The pressure released, and everyone began speaking at once. Those in the Group who were still smoking could now have greater self-respect as they saw their challenge through Clarence's struggle. As smokers, we can belittle ourselves with the self-judgment that quitting shouldn't be so hard. Seeing what Clarence was going through—Clarence, who had for years been perceived as strong and invincible—gave the Group a new basis for self-respect. If it was hard for him, it was no surprise that it was difficult for others to gain freedom from smoking. People who were smoke-free spoke of the need never to take being smoke-free for granted. We began to explore together what needed to be in place to keep ourselves away from cigarettes during difficult times, and we agreed that it is critically important to learn how to ask for help when we need it.

Over years of not smoking, Clarence had built a new life for himself. By quitting smoking, he'd "gotten real." He found and experienced who he *really* was and could be without cigarettes. He had the energy to enjoy his grandsons. (In the photo of Clarence in Chapter Eight, you can see his stacks of medical records from before [tall] and after [short] he quit smoking.) He also touched many lives, both in his work as a peer smoking-cessation counselor and in the work he did for disabled seniors.

Soon after telling the Group that he was smoking, and within months of relapsing, Clarence was found in a little sitting area outside of his house. Sometime the evening before, his body had died. His great spirit continues on as a loving and powerful example to all who get to hear his story.

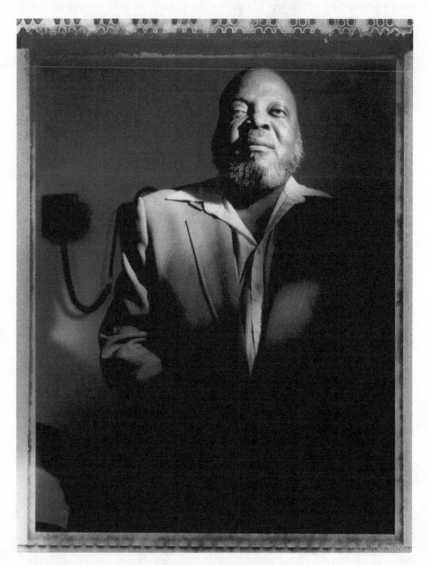

Clarence Brown   Photo by John Harding

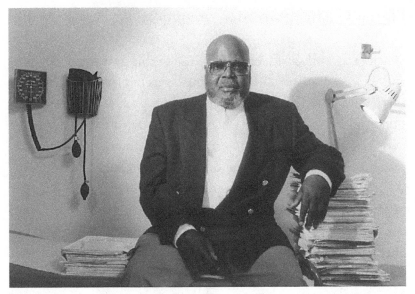

Clarence and his stacks of medical records from before *(on the right)* and after *(on the left)* he quit smoking.

Photo by John Harding

Clarence Brown, in His Own Voice

When I was working in the shipyard, all the big guys, the supervisor, and the best draftsmen were smoking cigars or cigarettes. They said they could think better. So I bought me a pack of Viceroys. Next thing you know, I find that when I start getting stressful, I want to have a cigarette. When I'm in a happy mood and want to celebrate, I want to have a cigarette. So now I got the nicotine addiction.

In 1959, I was diagnosed with sarcoid [an inflammatory disease of the organs]. I had started working for these record companies. Man, I'd be in the recording studio with two boxes of Shermans. We'd be sitting at that control panel, and by lunchtime, one box would be empty.

I really started having problems in 1979. I was diagnosed with asthma. Shit, everybody told me not to smoke. It didn't mean nothin'. After a while, you can say "I know it's killing me, but I'm gonna quit one day." "Yeah, I'm gonna quit next year." "I'm gonna quit smoking on my twenty-fifth birthday." "Well, no, I think I'll wait until I am forty." Oh, I know it's bad for me, but I'm going to die of something anyhow."

It was when I was working for the record companies that I started using heroin. It begins with the heroin to go to sleep at night. And then one day you find that in the morning you need a little snort to get the kinks out of your bones, and then the cocaine—zoom—gets you going. But I decided, man, this don't make sense, because I felt [using these substances] had something to do with my respiratory system. When I kicked heroin, I kept smoking.

"When I kicked heroin, I kept smoking."

I was a fool burning up, I was smoking so much. I was smoking Camels at the time, about three packs a day. I'd be trying to breathe. I'd take me a little breathing treatment and then I'd turn right back around and light me a cigarette.

Even though you're in a self-destruct mode and you're ruining your life, you have a tendency to think, "Oh, I got control of my shit." But once you come out of that altered state of mind, you realize that you didn't have control of it. When you're out of the addiction, you start thinking healthy. In the Bible it says, "Keep thy tabernacle clean." It's saying your body is the tabernacle, and when you feed all this poison to your body, you can't care about it, because you're only destroying it. And it's not an instant destruction; it's gradual. Just like with drugs. At first you say "Oh, I'm cool, I'm cool, I ain't hooked, I'm cool, I'm cool ... Oh man, goddamn, I'm really hooked!"

"First, second, third, fourth, fifth time I was intubated, and no, I didn't quit smoking."

My health was terrible. Terrible. From 1981 to 1989, I was in the hospital a lot. During one year, I was admitted twelve different times. One month I was admitted three times, and the last time they intubated me. They put this tube down into my lungs—being as how I couldn't breathe myself—and I had to be on a life-support machine. First, second, third, fourth, fifth time I was intubated, and no, I didn't quit smoking. I didn't even think about it. About the sixth time, I said "Man, wait a minute: It's about time I started doing something." So I came to one of the smoking-cessation Groups. Then I came back again. I think I came back three or four times before I finally quit smoking. Quitting cigarettes was a hard, hard thing to do—much harder than heroin or cocaine because of the availability. You don't have to go to no strange means to obtain cigarettes. Being in Group with other smokers really helped me.

If you really, really have a desire to quit smoking, you've got to be willing to separate yourself from smokers for at least three months. If you're around a group of people and they're smoking, you are going to have a problem because you see so many people looking pleasurable, looking cool. Then that brain says, "Hey, man. It's all right to have that one cigarette." And there you go; you're back into it.

Cigarettes can put you into a mood. You can use smoking as a mind-altering, mood-changing addiction. You can be mad about something and then say, "Hey, gimme a cigarette," to get over it. But if you stopped and thought about what you were doing, you would know that you can relieve the anxiety and be healthier by just sitting there and deep breathing ten times. Deep breathing helped me tremendously. I use it a lot for a lot of different things now.

When you are getting off cigarettes, you begin to have healthier thoughts about things. One morning I woke up, looked in the mirror, and said, "Hey, old dude." So, now I've formed a relationship with that person to the point that when I wake up in the morning, I say "Morning, bro," and it has become a ritual. When I was in the process of quitting smoking, I even carried it a bit further. I'd go to that mirror and I'd say, "Good morning," and I'd stand there and talk to myself. I'd say, "Now you ain't gonna smoke today, you are not going to have no cigarettes today." It was like something I would program back into my subconscious mind.

I found it was strong support because I would sometimes flash back on my conversation in that mirror and the promises that I had made to myself. People think I'm crazy, they probably do, and I *am* a little crazy, but I think it's good. It's a way to start letting yourself know, "Hey, I can do it. Me."

You gotta get your grass green first. Because if you're not loving yourself or caring about yourself, you can't love nobody else, you can't trust nobody else. This is what I'm saying about my life. I lived life in a self-destruct mode. By not caring for *myself* and not loving *myself* enough to make myself healthy, and not being the person that I can be, I can't trust *you*. The world was full of shit. And down with the world. And everything was down. But the minute I started making my grass green, I looked out and I said,

"I don't want to feel like I used to feel, no way."

"Hey, all the grass out there ain't brown. There is some green grass out there." In life, you're always going to have spots of brown grass around. But if you cultivate it right, it can turn green.

I got all kinds of benefits from not smoking. Some were surprises. I got involved in doing some volunteer work. At first, I thought "Volunteer? Shit, who the hell wants to do volunteer work?" But before I knew it, I found myself volunteering. With more energy from not smoking, you have a tendency to try and do more things. Now I'm more active.

My family, they are rejoicing that I quit, and they even tell me that I ain't so grumpy or rude or nasty to folks. Used to be I didn't care if I was going to die tomorrow or if I was going to live to see my grandchildren grow up. Now they're like my little road dogs; they always want to hang with me, and I find a great sense of joy with them.

Shit, man, I don't want to feel like I used to feel, no way.

Who would Clarence Brown be without cigarettes?

By quitting smoking, Clarence gave himself the chance to live and breathe and feel better. Feeling better allowed his true generosity and charisma to emerge. He became a productive member of his community and a powerful protector of his family.

Motivation is what gets you started. Habit is what keeps you going. **Jim Ryun**

Bill Johnson

Bill is a former drug addict who is a substance-abuse counselor. He has the self-awareness of someone who has been practicing sobriety for many years. Because he understands the power of addiction, he approached overcoming smoking methodically and with determination.

A pale, thin, serious man, Bill has tattoos covering his arms, and his white hair reaches down to the middle of his back. Short on words, he is shy, quiet, and a good listener. He would appear at Group with books under his arm, many of which were relevant to his study of addiction. Bill applied what he had learned in 12-step programs to stopping smoking, and he quickly achieved success. Because of his familiarity with making amends (step eight), he found a particularly meaningful use for the money he saved by not buying cigarettes. As you will read in his story, his decision to become smoke-free changed his life in a rich and surprising way.

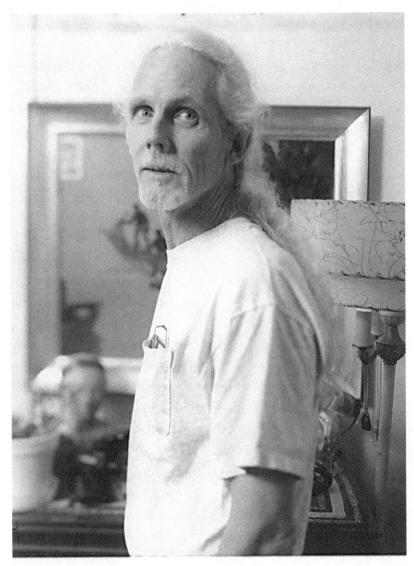

Bill Johnson

Photo by John Harding

Bill Johnson, in His Own Voice

My dad had a ninth-grade education. He's from the slums of Chicago; so is my mother. When he was young, Dad hitchhiked out West because there were too many poor kids trying to get into the military in Chicago. He joined the army in Colorado in 1935 and stayed in the military until 1960.

My father died of lung cancer when he was 56. He was a smoker. He smoked Lucky Strikes; a couple packs a day.

I started smoking. I drank alcohol and did other things like that when I was thirteen. I was a regular smoker by ninth grade. On the army base, a pack of cigarettes cost about 25 cents out of a machine. Any kid could buy cigarettes. It was never a problem for me getting cigarettes; and, for a long time, I didn't have the sense that I was hooked.

In the eighth grade, I broke my arm. I was in the military hospital on a ward with a bunch of Marines. Marines like kids, and these guys were giving me Camel cigarettes and looking after me. I remember smoking a lot. I also started to be nervous, around that time of my life. It had a lot to do with cigarettes and alcohol.

For me, tobacco was what, today, you'd call a gateway drug. When I was eighteen, I started using other drugs. I started smoking pot, I took bennies, I sniffed glue. After I got out of school, I started using acid and speed; then I started shooting speed and then barbiturates and heroin. I was a heroin addict for 27 years. I smoked all through that period; from the time I was in the ninth grade, it was normal for me to have a cigarette as soon as I got out of bed.

I was homeless and poor for a long time. I would collect butts off the street and break them down and roll the tobacco in Zig-Zags. I would steal cigarettes. I would bum cigarettes; I would embarrass myself to get a cigarette. I smoked and coughed, and I couldn't stop. The turning point was my throat hurting all the time; I was afraid I was going to get cancer and die like my father did. I saw my father have one lung removed and his larynx cut and not be able to speak for the last year of his life. He was in his fifties and going to college, a man with a ninth-grade education going to college; and he wiped out in a year.

Cigarettes were the last of my addictions that I got clean from. It took me a long time to quit smoking, even when I wanted to. It was very stressful. When I quit smoking the first time, I relapsed on heroin—that's how stressful it was. I didn't know how to talk about or take care of myself in my early sobriety. I became very irritable and agitated and unhappy and had a lot of mood swings. I lost my temper a lot; I had to really watch what I was doing. When I had my relapse, I started smoking again. I was using heroin, and I would buy one cigarette so I could break the filter off to strain my heroin through it and then I would give the cigarette to a street person. But one time I took the cigarette with me where I went to fix; I broke the filter off to use the cotton; and I lit the cigarette. And that was it: I was right back up to a pack a day.

"Now my son calls me; he and I have a relationship."

When I was ready to quit again, I made a new plan. I stayed in Group longer, I did aftercare longer, and I intensified my work around my drug use. I got support, did things like celebrate every day, every milestone. Drinking a lot of water and jogging, and acupuncture really helped me too. Within six months of not smoking, my throat wasn't sore all the time.

In Group, we figured out how much [our habit] cost. I was divorced years ago and I never sent my kid any money. I was getting ready to make amends to my ex-wife, even though I hadn't seen her in years. I figured out I would have enough money to pay my child support, even though my son was a grown man. Since I quit smoking 31 months ago, I've been sending my ex-wife $50 a month.

Quitting smoking has allowed me to be more responsible, to take something bad out of my life and replace it with something good. Now my son calls me; he and I have a relationship. He came out here to see me after years of never seeing him. Who ever thought that quitting smoking would help me pay my child support and give me back my son?

Who would Bill Johnson be without cigarettes?

For decades, Bill used cigarettes as a means of maintaining control. By becoming a non-smoker, Bill achieved real self-control and uncovered qualities about himself that changed his life: he became more responsible, as shown by his decision to start paying child support. And he became a more caring and committed parent, which finally allowed him to enjoy a relationship with his son.

What can we gain by sailing to the moon if we are not able to cross the abyss that separates us from ourselves? This is the most important of all voyages of discovery. **Thomas Merton**

Mary Nordseth

Mary's quiet intensity and gentle humor covered a complex character and history that slowly attracted the interest of the Group: who *was* this woman? As it turned out, she was in a deep process of self-discovery, and becoming a part of the Group was a significant part of her growing commitment to herself. We in the Group were getting to know her as she was getting to know herself.

When Mary first joined our Group, she was watchful and quiet. As she listened and observed, I could tell she was trying to see if she could trust us. Before much time passed, she stepped in and began practicing a ruthless honesty, primarily allowing us to overhear her own inner dialogue about what she had been doing with her life and why. In the environment of authenticity and truth-telling that characterized the Group, she seemed to find the courage she needed to begin uncovering secrets she had been keeping from herself.

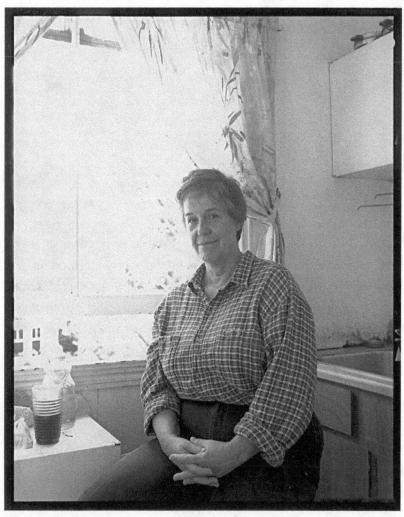

Mary Nordseth   Photo by John Harding

Mary Nordseth, in Her Own Voice

I was born in the East Bay. By the time I was in the tenth grade, my parents were divorced. I quit high school and went to work to support my brother, sister, mother, and myself. I was sixteen. I continued to do this until my mother remarried, and then I moved to San Francisco at twenty-one.

I never saw my mother without a cigarette, never. When she would get ready to go out, I was the little attendant, and I would hold the cigarette for her. I would make a big deal about how I hated it. I started smoking when I was fourteen.

People who have emphysema are literally trying to suck air in through their skin. That was my mother. She died ten years ago. I was told that her lungs were so black, they didn't know if she had lung cancer. So, I knew what smoking could do to a person, but it didn't stop me. I smoked two packs a day.

In 1964, the first *Surgeon General's Report on Smoking and Health* came out, and I had a little twinge of conscience. But nothing was going to make me quit smoking. It was part of my image, the wise guy, the person who had everything under control. I couldn't step back far enough to see what I was doing to myself until I got in a group of people who could hold my hand. Only then could I look at the damage not only to my body but also to my ambition. I was choosing something that was killing me. I had destroyed the quality of my life. Smoking affected the direction of my life. I was a very athletic kid; I'd gotten free tennis lessons because I had such ability. In the 1960s, I'd go to Big Sur with friends. Everyone but me would get out of the car. I would sit and have a cigarette. But that wasn't really who I was. Smoking

"I never saw my mother without a cigarette, never."

changed who I was; it changed the direction of my life. It changed the very person I might have become.

I got hooked shooting methedrine and then heroin. I was a very heavy marijuana smoker. If I had not started smoking, I wouldn't have taken drugs; the cigarettes paved the way. I could never really look at my problems directly because I could always step aside and put these chemicals into my body to distract myself from whatever they were. It's really sad what cigarettes have done to people.

The cessation program gave me the opportunity to look at myself, first, through the eyes of other people. I did not have their honesty; I borrowed from them. People were really talking the truth, and I wished I could be that honest, be that in touch with myself, and really speak from my heart. I could not speak from my heart because I didn't know what my feelings were. I wanted that honesty and that connection with my own feelings that I saw from so many people there. In a hopeless situation, the Group offered hope.

> "Once the tobacco and chemicals were withdrawn, I was free to be more of who I am."

I was stilted emotionally from the cigarettes. My emotions were locked up. Once the tobacco and chemicals were withdrawn, I was free to be more of who I am. Emotions are connected with the person I had not been in touch with for a very long time. My emotions came to the surface, and as I spread my feelings around, I found there were feelings for everybody in that class. I had to find something that was stronger than me, and in the beginning, it was the Group. The cessation Group was the part of me that I had lost touch with, that part of me that really cared about me. It was the person that I had lost who said, "This is dangerous," or, "Have you noticed you have to stop walking up your steps when you're going home with your groceries?" Each time, everyone had something to offer; and I could take some of that with me in those moments when I felt uncertain and afraid of relapsing. The class was my support.

"I owe 75 percent of my success in quitting cigarettes to exercise."

I had very strong withdrawal, tremendous anxiety—like an exaggerated grief—because I can't have what I want. The only way I could get over it was to wear myself out, hiking. I owe 75 percent of my success in quitting cigarettes to exercise. It helps generate endorphins in the body; it helps me sweat, and that cleansing is so important. I put all my energy into exercising and cleaning my system.

A cigarette is a controlling tool. When a person frees up to [acknowledge] his or her own needs and wants, life is more fluid. If I say something stupid or I make a faux pas, I don't grieve over it the way I did when I was a smoker; I just go on. There's more fluidity. Everything is lighter. That fluidity comes from being in touch with my feelings. *Emotion* is just what the word says: it's *motion,* it's movement. I let myself be drawn by my feelings. Being in touch with my feelings is the greatest gift I've gotten from quitting cigarettes.

I don't want to smoke anymore. I don't have to. How simple, and yet what a long journey to get to that place.

Who would Mary Nordseth be without cigarettes?

Mary quit smoking and became more honest and truthful, qualities that were deeply important to her. The process of becoming smoke-free gave her the opportunity to practice self-investigation. Living without cigarettes also allowed her to develop her natural poetic creativity.

All of humanity's problems stem from man's inability to sit quietly in a room alone. **Blaise Pascal**

Pete Anastole

Pete's body was a bundle of thumps and vibrations. During his first year in the program, he came sporadically to Group and was so agitated that, by the end of the hour, he had sat in nearly every empty chair in the room. When he did stop and sit, he drummed his fingers incessantly on the tabletop while furiously pumping one foot up and down. A furniture mover by trade, Pete is a large, burly, handsome man. He would sometimes show up to Group with his girlfriend, and both would have bruises on their arms from their fights with each other.

After more than a year of dropping in and out of Group, Pete finally decided to commit fully to quit smoking. To help control his withdrawal symptoms, he chose to use a nicotine patch. But he ended up wearing it for no more than a few hours before he ripped it off his body in disgust: he was "not going to rely on any crutch."

What followed were some of the worst withdrawals I have ever witnessed in a smoker. Pete admitted to throwing heavy objects across the room and even out the window. He huddled, shaking and sweating, under the bed covers for days. When he appeared in Group with bruises on his face and arms, I was alarmed to learn of the battering that resulted when the fights with his girlfriend escalated. A couple of weeks later, when he reported that they had broken up, I was flooded with relief.

Over the next few weeks, I watched as Pete's agitation continued to build. He was impatient and jumpy in Group and generally felt miserable. It wasn't until he began to increase his level of exercise and cut back on coffee and other caffeinated drinks that his demeanor began to shift. Soon, he was able to sit in one chair for an entire hour; his drumming on the table lessened and, then stopped altogether. Within a few months, Pete was actually able to listen to other Group members and share the skills and experience he had learned on his journey.

Pete continued to participate in Group over several years. He grew calmer and more centered, losing many of his former signs of agitation and discomfort in his own skin, of the tension that had characterized him as a smoker. Increasingly self-aware, he decided to learn how to manage his angry feelings and joined a program for men overcoming violence. With the insights he gained from facing his inner demons, Pete developed into an accomplished, thoughtful, and compassionate peer counselor, guiding and supporting other smokers to a smoke-free life. He continued exercising and began to address his diet, lowering the large amount of simple sugars and carbohydrates that had been staples for him. Quitting smoking ultimately led to serenity and relaxation and cultivated strong leadership qualities that he used to help others who were where he had once been.

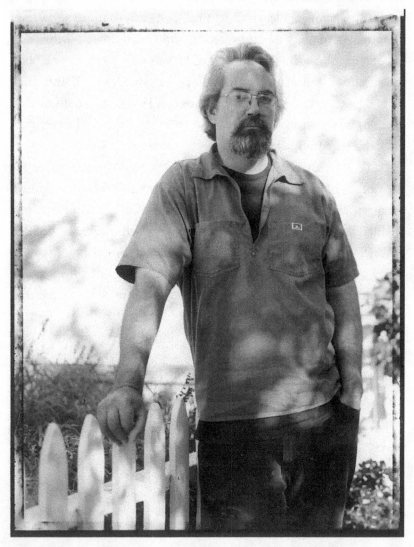

Pete Anastole

Photo by Greene and Harding

Pete Anastole, in His Own Voice

Everybody in the house smoked. Everybody. My mother smoked four packs a day; my father would smoke two packs. My uncle, who was over all the time, smoked four packs a day. So right there, you are looking at ten packs of cigarettes a day being smoked in a small, one-bedroom house. My nose ran twenty-four hours a day. I always had a cold, I always coughed. I began smoking by stealing the butts my uncle threw out the window. I was ten years old.

Around the ninth grade, I started smoking a pack a day. I made it my mission to smoke, and within two weeks, I was hooked on cigarettes. I liked the rush that smoking gave me. From then on, it was downhill.

I was a big man. Size gives you a kind of power. People who were your enemies are now your friends, and they want to bum cigarettes. Your peers gave you more respect because you were a smoker. At fourteen, fifteen, sixteen years old, you rule the world, and you don't think about anything. But after a while, I discovered I couldn't walk long distances.

In my early thirties, I was in the moving business, and I was tired all the time. I was smoking two to two-and-a-half packs a day. If I had five dollars in my pocket and I was starving, and it was buy food or buy cigarettes, I would buy cigarettes. I was irritated all the time, ready to fight at the drop of a hat. My nervousness was uncontrollable, my outbreaks of anger steady. Guys who were fifty years old were running past me.

The realization of death—the knowledge that you are going to die if you don't stop doing smoking—is

> "If I had five dollars in my pocket and I was starving, and it was buy food or buy cigarettes, I would buy cigarettes."

what did it for me. My brother and I, we walked a mile and a half in pouring rain. I was out of breath and we had to go down a big hill. If I had gone all the way to the bottom, I would have never come back up, so I couldn't go down there and be with him. He said, "What are you going to do three or four years from now? You won't even get out of the car. You will be hooked up to an oxygen bottle and pointing your finger." That's when I said to myself, "I'd better do something about this smoking. Each individual has the power to change, so I am going to use that power to change."

The first time I went to Group, I went for two weeks. A year and a half later, I went back again. This time, I went further into the Group and then I said, "Well, I can't quit, something is wrong," and left. The third time, I made a no-smoking zone in the truck. I wouldn't let anyone smoke in the truck. I would pull over, park, get out, smoke, put the cigarette out, and get back in. Pretty soon, I would make it from my house to work without stopping, so I eliminated one or two cigarettes on the way to work. After a while, I was able to extend the time without a cigarette. At the end of the class, I quit.

I suffered all that day. I stayed in bed and shook like a junkie kicking heroin. I was sweating, I was pulling the covers over my head, and I was screaming and yelling. It was a living hell—the worst seven days of my life. I had never done anything that hard. It was a great personal accomplishment; I had reached an important crossroads.

All of my life, I had an anger issue. I didn't know what to do with my anger. It was always inside looking for somewhere to go, so I released it onto people I loved. I would get mad and abuse women. I was mad all the time. I never had a grip on how to handle anger; I was always upset at or about someone. When I quit smoking, I had to deal with my anger because I had no more vices to control it with. Now I face my anger, and by facing it, I feel calmer, more at ease. I put everything in perspective. Before, I would worry about something small, like missing a bus. I would quickly lose control and then fall into a major depression behind it. Now I say to myself, "Okay, I missed the bus, so go get some coffee and sit and relax." Or I go out for a walk and do some deep breathing and I calm down.

I give myself no more than thirty minutes to be angry about an issue, and then I say to myself, "Okay, 30 minutes are up; it's time to move on to something else." There's stuff I would dwell on every day, and because I knew I couldn't let it consume me anymore, I would try to put it to the side. Being able to do this takes practice, but the more you do it, the better you are going to get at it. Before, I never let anybody get a word in. Now I will sit and listen; I notice [when] people say things I can use. I am learning stuff about myself that I never knew existed. I am open to new ideas, different ways of approaching things.

So much time is consumed smoking fifty cigarettes a day: smoke, exhale, put it out, don't burn your clothes, buy more cigarettes before you run out. Two to three hours of the day are eaten up this way, so that is two to three hours a day that I have gained. I like nature, so I started walking in parks, places that I never would have stopped to look at before. Walking gave me a sense of progress. I could walk up a couple of hills the first week. After a while, I could go up three, four, five hills without stopping. I tried changing my diet to more fruits and vegetables. I drank a lot of water. The money I save from not smoking I am going to put down on my own piece of property. That's five acres in the country that the tobacco company can't have. They are mine. The tobacco people will take everything you've got.

"After a while, I could go up three, four, five hills without stopping."

I didn't expect the withdrawal to be as strong as it was, I didn't expect the anger and emotion to come to the extreme height that they did, and I didn't expect to feel as good as I do right now. I have my life back, my personal dignity. I can work. I can walk two and a half miles every day. I am becoming more self-aware. I feel so much self-respect because I was able to take control of something that was controlling my life and put it aside. I am learning how to deal with my problems that were always there but which I suppressed with cigarettes.

Use whatever you can. If you read, then read; if you walk, walk. Exercise and water are good. Use what you can to get the nicotine out of your body. Keep your mind occupied. You have to beat smoking or it will beat you. I have been to a lot of funerals for folks who smoked.

Who would Pete Anastole be without cigarettes?

Once he was no longer using cigarettes to suppress his anger, Pete was free to confront his feelings and learn to use emotional energy as a productive force. He relaxed into himself and became more integrated and connected with people in his life.

Who would you be without cigarettes?

Action steps for people who want to be smoke-free

During the years that he worked to stop smoking, Clarence explored and experimented with a variety of skills. The single most important practice he found that helped him to stop smoking and stay smoke-free was deep abdominal breathing. At first, Clarence used this relaxation technique to eliminate stress-related cigarettes: instead of reaching for a cigarette, he would take five slow, deep breaths, fully expanding his abdomen. After becoming smoke-free, he continued to rely on this practice whenever he felt an urge for a cigarette.

Try taking deep abdominal breaths regularly. At first, practice when you are *not* under stress or facing a strong urge, because when you are in the middle of a crisis, it will be too difficult to learn a new behavior. If you were going to run a marathon (and stopping smoking can be compared to such a challenge), you would invest time in building strength, stamina, and endurance. You wouldn't just show up on the day of the marathon and expect to do well without any training. The same is true of the stress-management tool of deep breathing: **the skill will be there when you need it if you practice during times when you aren't facing stressful feelings.** Once you have learned the skill, you can use it whenever you have the urge to smoke. To begin, imagine you are blowing out candles on a birthday cake; take in a breath before blowing out all the air you can, and then allow a deep breath to come in naturally. Repeat this five times.

Clarence liked the skills he could easily integrate into a daily routine. For example, each morning he'd look into his own eyes in the bathroom mirror and make himself a promise: Speaking out loud, he'd declare, "Dude, I'm gonna take care of you today; it's gonna be a smoke-free day." Then, during the day, when he had an urge to smoke, he'd remember his promise and feel strong in his decision. For all the years he remained a non-smoker, Clarence did not scare himself with thoughts of "I can never again have a cigarette." Instead, he took it one day at a time, making a promise for that day only. Thinking that you can never have another cigarette in your whole life can be enough to send at least some of us desperately reaching for a smoke. Instead, try focusing on the present: "For right now, I'm smoke-free. For the next hour or the next day, I'm going to breathe fresh, clean air." Measuring your journey in small increments makes it less overwhelming and more likely that you can sustain yourself through the long haul.

Each person in this chapter used smoking to manage or suppress his or her feelings. Ironically, while smoking helped them to keep some emotional control in their lives, it ultimately controlled them. Stopping smoking gave them the chance to turn weakness into strength. The process of getting smoke-free demanded that they look at aspects of themselves that they had been avoiding with cigarettes. Pete used cigarettes to control anger. To become truly free, he had to look at his anger directly and find healthy ways to manage it. As he consciously explored and examined his anger, he learned to be more focused and calm. Barbara got in touch with feelings she had avoided, including the uneasiness she felt about how smoking worsened her breathing symptoms. In learning to express her natural emotions, she found that her life was enriched because she could experience feelings more completely.

> "Although you most likely have an idea of what health benefits you will enjoy by quitting smoking, there is no way to predict what other gifts you will receive."

Although you most likely have an idea of what health benefits you will enjoy by quitting smoking, there is no way to predict what other gifts you will receive. If you try to look at what you're most afraid of about quitting, you might find a clue about what new strengths may become available to you. For example, some people are afraid of overeating and gaining weight. If this is true for you, how could you meet that fear directly and creatively? Perhaps you'll want to experiment with cooking light or with making delicious low-calorie snacks. You may find that letting go of cigarettes will spur you to have a healthier relationship with food. What might that look like?

You might also be anxious about feeling bored or sad or angry. If boredom is an issue for you, try to come up with some unexplored interests. Boredom is a state out of which creativity is born. What is something you've been putting off, thinking you might do some day? What about learning to play the piano or knit or to do Sudoku puzzles? Or maybe you've always wanted to study Italian. It's hard to be bored when you're doing something interesting.

If sadness is an issue, think about what gives you pleasure and makes you happy. Does being in nature lift your spirits? You and a friend might enjoy planning day trips to beautiful places near where you live. If anger is an issue, getting more exercise can help tremendously. Starting an exercise program doesn't have to be complicated: you can begin with walking ten to thirty minutes a day and build from there.

Exercise is an effective way to release some of the uncomfortable feelings of withdrawal. It also helps to counter weight gain. How can you increase the amount of exercise you are getting? Simple things like getting off the bus a few stops before your destination can make a difference. Making a pact

> Take a few minutes to jot down some ideas about what you have been avoiding by smoking and what you might be interested in exploring or practicing as a non-smoker.

with a friend to take an exercise class together or going dancing on a regular basis are other fun options that provide support and companionship.

Take a few minutes to jot down some ideas about what you have been avoiding by smoking and what you might be interested in exploring or practicing as a non-smoker. Consider for a moment: who might you be without cigarettes? What difference might that change make in your life and in the lives of others around you? Then be prepared for some wonderful surprises once you get through the uncomfortable transition period of becoming smoke-free.

Three Key Points

1. Tobacco dependence can keep us emotionally frozen at the developmental stage we were in when we first started smoking.

2. Smoking blocks us from developing effective coping skills for everyday life.

3. Becoming smoke-free gives us the opportunity to experience and express a wider emotional range, making life ultimately more authentic and fulfilling.

NOTES

CHAPTER NINE

Changing How We Think and What We Do: Tips and Skills to Become a Non-Smoker

Note: You might recognize some of the information here from other chapters. We think it's important to collect it here, in one place.

What we think has everything to do with what actions we take. This chapter will explore ways to harness the power of your mind to support the changes you have worked to accomplish. On the journey to becoming a non-smoker, there is one truth that can help steady you through the ups and downs: every cigarette you don't smoke counts. Saying "Every cigarette I don't smoke counts" to yourself helps to keep you from going back to regular smoking if you slip up. It can also give you something to hold on to when urges arise and when you are in difficult situations.

Many of us find it reassuring to count the cigarettes we didn't smoke. After just one month, the number of unsmoked cigarettes for a pack-a-day smoker would be 600! Picturing that stack reinforces your success. And if you go for a few days or weeks and slip up, counting the cigarettes you did *not* smoke can keep you out of the pit of thinking "I'm a failure and may as well smoke."

> "Many of us find it reassuring to count the cigarettes we didn't smoke."

Let's begin our exploration by looking at motivation: what it is and how it works.

Motivation

Motivation often happens in response to the feeling that things are not how we want or think they should be. When we are not comfortable with how things are, we look for the energy to take action and get things back to normal. You come home after a long day at work to discover the kitchen pipes have burst. You're tired, wanting to crash on the couch and watch TV. But those pipes have to be fixed, and your energy arises to deal with the problem. You spring into action to get things back to normal. That's motivation in action.

When you work to change your behavior, take advantage of motivational energy whenever you can. Otherwise, the energy will fade, and you'll have missed a chance to use it for change. Remember the example of remodeling your house. The rooms are painted and the only thing left to do is to install the switch plates over the light switches. For days, you'll notice the holes, and this last chore will nag at you. However, if you let enough time go by, you will get used to those holes. It could be weeks or months—or never—before you finally take care of this last detail.

If you want to stop smoking, notice whenever something motivates you—unpleasant feelings, a desire to be smoke-free— and then find ways to take advantage of that energy to change. You might skip the next few cigarettes, join a group or an online forum dedicated to stopping smoking, or take a trip to the store and buy a package of colorful star stickers to mark every smoke-free day on a special calendar. Your response can be even simpler: take five deep breaths while picturing yourself becoming calm and centered. Actions like these will build energy to carry you toward your smoke-free goal. You don't have to wait for motivation to arise. You can actively grow the motivation to change.

"You don't have to wait for motivation to arise."

Fear-Based and Desire-Based Motivation

Two basic kinds of motivation exist: fear-based and desire-based. When it comes to quitting, we feel plenty of fear-based motivations. Doctors, nurses, friends, and family may describe dire consequences of what will happen if we keep smoking: "Mr. Brown, if you don't stop smoking immediately, you are going to kill yourself." Or, "Daddy, I don't want you to die; please stop smoking." Such messages can trigger so much worry that we want to smoke to manage our discomfort. While it is normal to be defensive—"You're not my boss," "I smoke because I like it," "I'll stop whenever I please"—sometimes that defense might be hiding the fear that you can't quit. In reaction, we defensively do more of whatever we're being told to change.

> "Such messages can trigger so much worry that we want to smoke to manage our discomfort."

Fear restricts behavior: avoiding one thing and doing something else that "I *have* to do." Who wants to do what we *have* to do or what we *should* do? We feel weak, powerless, hopeless, stuck, and even worthless. When I worked on a cancer unit and was faced with daily reminders of the dreadful things that could happen if I kept smoking, my fear led me to smoke more to deal with the anxiety. And my smoking kept the fear alive. Every puff disturbed me.

When it comes to changing unhealthy behaviors, the only positive side of fear is that it can snap us out of denial. For example, if you developed persistent throat pain that led to the need for medical tests, you might be shocked enough to quit smoking. But trying to beat yourself into change by telling yourself scary stories about what *could* happen will weaken you, increasing your feelings of powerlessness and worthlessness. These feelings don't help successful behavior change.

On the other hand, *desire*-based motivation can help to get you moving. People like to go after what they want. If someone pushes you to do something, you might dig in your heels and resist. However, you will willingly follow something you want. Desire-based motivation puts us back in control; it encourages action and sets us in motion to succeed. Following our desires builds confidence. We feel strong and empowered and hopeful. Being motivated by desire supports self-worth and gives us the feeling of having choices. Most important, desire-based motivation helps create lasting change.

> "Desire-based motivation puts us back in control; it encourages action and sets us in motion to succeed."

If you didn't do it while reading the last chapter, take a moment and try this experiment. Put down this book, close your eyes, and allow your mind to quiet as you follow your breath coming in and out of your body. Now, in your mind or out loud, say, "I *have* to stop smoking, I *have* to stop smoking." Repeat this phrase a few times, and as you do, feel the urgency in your words. Notice your body sensations and any thoughts or feelings that happen. What do you feel as you repeat, "I *have* to stop smoking"? Take a minute or two to jot down a few words to describe your experience.

Now, closing your eyes again, say, "I *want* to stop smoking." Even if part of you does not believe this is true, repeat it while imagining that it is what you truly want. Say the phrase a few times as you think about any body sensations and thoughts and feelings. What do you notice? Take another moment to record your thoughts.

Participants report that when they say "I have to ... ," they feel tightness. Sometimes there is a feeling of panic or a sense of hopelessness. Your mind says "*no*, I don't" or "but I can't." On the other hand, repeating "I want to ... " results in feelings of openness and choice. You feel relaxed and think, "It's my choice, and I can do it."

The important thing to remember, when looking at these two kinds of motivations, is that what you say to yourself in your own head is even more important than what gets said to you by others. Smokers attempt to abuse themselves into stopping by saying, "Why am I so stupid? I've *got* to stop smoking." In this way, they set up a battle between the part that says "I have to" and the part that says "I won't; I don't want to." This split makes it so much more difficult to move forward. It is like trying to drive with the brakes on.

Exercise: Your "Want To" (Desire-Based) Motivations

In our programs, one of the most important steps we ask people to take is to begin keeping a list of their "want to" motivations. We ask them to think about and write down why they want to stop smoking rather than why they *have to* stop. Sometimes it is easier to uncover what we want through deciding what we do *not* want. When I was stopping smoking, I knew that two of my most important reasons for wanting to be smoke-free were that I was struggling with fear and with feeling low self-esteem as a mother and a nurse. My fear was about whatever I might be doing to my future and myself by smoking. I also feared the challenge of stopping smoking. Every cigarette I smoked fueled fear, and when I wasn't actually smoking, the fearful atmosphere persisted. And smoking was not helping me be the best mother I could be. Plus, I saw myself as a negative role model for my patients, coming to their bedside reeking of cigarettes. Bottom line, my smoking made me both scared and ashamed.

> "I want to be fearless and proud."

Turning "I don't want to be afraid and guilty" into what I *did* want became "I want to be fearless and proud." I gave my attention to imagining what it would feel like to be fearless and proud. How would I hold my body as I experienced those feelings? What thoughts would I cultivate? I practiced fearlessness and pride and made little signs to put up around my house and in my car that read, "I am smoke-free, fearless, and proud." In this way, I slowly reprogrammed myself to feel what I *wanted* to be true. This reprogramming became the powerful support guiding and sustaining me through withdrawal symptoms and challenging situations as I rebuilt my life as a non-smoker.

It is hard enough to quit smoking without getting into a battle with yourself. A key step is to *join your own team*. Don't berate yourself for not being what you think you should be. Instead, encourage yourself with positive thoughts. Take a moment and experiment with a powerful exercise. On a piece of paper, start a list of your personal reasons for wanting to be smoke-free. Keep adding to this list over the next days and weeks, building a foundation for embracing the new life you are creating.

Use Language to Support Your Efforts to Stop Smoking

The things we believe strongly influence what we do. If I believe that I need cigarettes to deal with stress, when faced with stress, I will automatically reach for a cigarette. With this direct connection between belief and action, it's worthwhile to identify and change beliefs to support new behavior.

Language gives us the most direct access to changing beliefs. What you tell yourself shapes what you do. Using clear, goal-focused language, you can override negative feelings and thoughts that don't align with the results you want. The following two ways of thinking about stopping smoking lead to very different results:

1. In the first perspective, you tell yourself you are being denied something you love: *Something I want/need has been taken away from me. Why should I have to suffer? I feel so sorry for myself.... I have lost my best friend! I really want to*

smoke.... It should not be this hard! Why can't I smoke every once in a while? I really hate this.

Not surprisingly, this way of thinking quickly leads back to smoking.

2. On the other hand, telling yourself you can do something has a more successful outcome: *This is an amazing opportunity for me to change. I am learning to deal with life without harming myself. Withdrawal symptoms are my body's way of healing from cigarettes. It is exciting to see that I am more powerful than cigarettes. This is the most important challenge I have ever taken on.*

This second way of thinking, a positive vision of being smoke-free, puts you on the road to your smoke-free goal. By repeating the beliefs you *want* to be true, you begin to replace old, negative beliefs with your new, positive outcomes.

Experiment with the impact of language. Start using positive, smoke-free language even if it sounds odd, fake, or like a lie. Four of the most powerful words you can say to yourself (even if it isn't quite true yet) are **I am smoke-free.** Take a moment here and refer back to your list of desires for being smoke-free. Choose one to three items that are especially important to you. Make a statement about being smoke-free using your chosen item(s).

Your statement will be most effective if you load it with words that have deep, personal meaning for you. For me, I wanted to feel *fearless* and *proud*. Beginning twenty-one days before my stop date, I repeated over and over to myself, "I am smoke-free, fearless, and proud." Not only did I write those words on sticky notes and paste them all over my home and in my car, but I also went to sleep at night muttering them. And in the morning when I woke up, I started saying them. They began to have more reality for me until, once I actually put out my last cigarette, I found that I had programmed myself to feel the truth I had chosen for myself. When urges came, I met them with my personal smoke-free mantra and felt positively relieved.

Another time to examine your use of language is when you describe your efforts to change. Many people

> "Using the word try leaves you with a way out."

say they are going to "try to" stop smoking, perhaps "over the weekend." Using the word try leaves you with a way out. The word itself implies some doubt about the effectiveness of your efforts. By saying you are going to try, you allow for the possibility of failure and give yourself an easy out: "Well, I tried. I'm still a good person, a good patient, a good parent; I tried." And then you go back to smoking. Begin using language that expresses greater confidence and commitment: "I *am* stopping smoking." After all, you have put a lot of thought and work into this stop date.

Dependence on Tobacco

Changing how you think and act is key to stopping smoking. Many smokers say that cigarettes have been their best friends who are always there when times are tough or when there is something to celebrate. Smokers typically come into stop-smoking programs when that friendship or love affair has turned: the smoker feels trapped and/or sick. Understanding what has kept you in an unhealthy relationship (in this case, with tobacco) can be useful to finding a way to end the relationship. In our program, we look at four factors that keep smokers tobacco-dependent: the addictive drug, nicotine; the hand-mouth stimulations of smoking; deep breathing; and the psychological and emotional basis for smoking.

As you read about these four aspects of tobacco dependence, think about which ones are relevant for you. Rate each one on a scale of zero to ten, with zero being unimportant and ten being extremely important. Write your scores right here in the book. After you rate these factors, you can tailor your quit program to address the issues that keep you smoking.

1. Nicotine

Nicotine is a stimulating and relaxing drug, in easy-to-use single doses: cigarettes. Depending on how you smoke cigarettes (for example, long, deep drags or quick, short puffs), the upper or downer effects can be emphasized, making the effects of nicotine adaptable to many situations. For example, nicotine can lessen stress or uncomfortable feelings on one side and increase alertness and energy on the other.

Nicotine is nearly as addictive as heroin, and it's legal. The tobacco industry has bombarded us with images of satisfied smokers in all kinds of situations. In the United States, tobacco companies can't advertise as they used to. But there are still smokers in movies. Young people are targets of the cigarette industry and are constantly exposed to images of their favorite movie stars lighting up.

> "Nicotine is nearly as addictive as heroin, and it's legal."

Because people can still smoke in many situations, you are constantly faced with the opportunity to light up. And because tobacco companies make it seem like an acceptable form of behavior, it's harder to kick the habit. If smoking is something you do with most of your friends, it's going to be difficult to hang out with those friends and not smoke. Or if you smoke each morning in your car on the way to work, simply getting into your car can trigger the desire to smoke. In California, smokers report that the limitations on where they can smoke are helpful because so many places are now off limits. Even with these restrictions, and despite any feelings people may have about smoking, it's still largely seen as a normal activity. How would you perceive a group of workers outside their office taking a quick smoke break? You might feel sorry for them or glad that you don't have to do that. What would you think about that same group gathered outside injecting drugs into their arms? Would you be shocked and surprised? Why? Because even though we are not accustomed to seeing people injecting their narcotics in public, we *have* grown used to seeing smokers sucking smoke into their lungs. Although smoking kills nearly half of the people who use tobacco, we have been conditioned to see it as "normal" behavior.

How important is nicotine in your relationship with cigarettes? If it turns out that nicotine is a strong part of your tobacco dependence, you could consider using nicotine replacement therapy (NRT) or other oral medications to help you become smoke-free. Chapter Fourteen provides a comprehensive discussion of how nicotine affects your brain and why it's so intensely addictive. Chapter Fifteen is a review of the available medications that can reduce strong urges and help you quit successfully. Here is a test you can complete to help you understand your level of nicotine addiction. Mark your answers right here in the book.

Fagerstrom Test for Nicotine Dependence (FTND)

For step number 1, please read the questions below. For each question, check the box that best describes your response.

1. How soon after you wake up do you smoke your first cigarette?

 ◯ Within 5 minutes (3 points)
 ◯ 6–30 minutes (2 points)
 ◯ 31–60 minutes (1 point)
 ◯ After 60 minutes (0 points)

2. Do you find it difficult to refrain from smoking in places where it is forbidden, e.g., in church, at the library, in cinemas?

 ◯ Yes (1 point)
 ◯ No (0 points)

3. Which cigarette would you hate most to give up?

 ◯ The first one in the morning (1 point)
 ◯ Any other (0 points)

4. How many cigarettes per day do you smoke?

 ◯ 31 or more (3 points)
 ◯ 21–30 (2 points)
 ◯ 11–20 (1 point)
 ◯ 10 or fewer (0 points)

5. Do you smoke more frequently during the first hours after waking up than during the rest of the day?

 ◯ Yes (1 point)
 ◯ No (0 points)

6. Do you smoke when you are so ill that you are in bed most of the day? (If you never get sick, give the most likely response.)

 ◯ Yes (1 point)
 ◯ No (0 points)

Scoring: Add up your points for each answer. For example, in Question 1, the answer "6–30 minutes" is worth two points.

5 points or more shows a significant dependence.

4 points or fewer show low to moderate dependence on nicotine.

Download a printable version at **www.learningtoquit.com/resources**.

2. The Hand-Mouth Stimulations of Smoking

By the time they get around to learning how to quit, most people have been smokers for years. This means they have repeated hand and mouth gestures thousands of times, and these actions have become habits when they smoke. Whether you: use a lighter or matches; tap the pack to pop up your next smoke or pull it out of the box; hold the cigarette between your thumb and index finger or between your index and middle fingers; smoke from the middle of your lips or from the corner of the mouth, all of these smoking behaviors are woven into the rewarding effects of nicotine. These movements and gestures are part of your unique signature of smoking dependence patterns and have grown into a part of the personal satisfaction and expression you get from smoking. Stopping smoking means the loss of all this hand, mouth, and visual activity.

During many of my own early attempts at quitting, I found myself overeating whenever I stopped smoking, quickly adding uncomfortable pounds. I told myself "Obviously I can't keep eating like this. I'll get as big as a barn. I have to smoke." It took a few rounds of this self-defeating relapse cycle before I committed myself to writing a different ending to my helplessness story. Strategies included putting a reasonable

"Stopping smoking means the loss of all this hand, mouth, and visual activity."

amount of food on my plate and, when I finished, pushing myself away from the table, going outside, walking around the block three or four times, and then returning home to wash the dishes. I also temporarily stopped eating cake, candy, and cookies and found that the cravings for sugary sweets stopped within about three days. Following this routine, my weight stopped increasing and my mood became more balanced. Like many people stopping smoking, I began to improve other health habits.

Even with these adjustments, I still needed to keep my hands busy, so I got creative. I started sculpting with porcelain clay and spent the next two years making life-size dolls. Then I discovered a love for painting, which has given me much greater satisfaction and freedom than cigarettes ever could. And I still light candles and incense to enjoy the beautiful patterns made by smoke as it swirls through the air.

3. Deep Breathing

One reason people smoke is that it requires them to take deep breaths—an action that is inherently satisfying. Our bodies are built to ensure that oxygen levels do not fall below what is necessary for healthy function. Of all the organs in the body, the brain has the greatest need for oxygen. When oxygen levels in the brain fall, we yawn or sigh, automatically bringing in a deeper breath. This natural impulse is hijacked by smoking,. When you would naturally yawn or sigh, you reach for a cigarette, light up, and take a deep drag.

> "Deep abdominal breathing is a simple and powerful tool to decrease stress and tension."

When I interviewed Clarence Brown after he stopped smoking, I asked him what tools had been most helpful in stopping successfully. Without hesitation he replied, "deep breathing." Deep abdominal breathing is a simple and powerful tool to decrease stress and tension.

Every cell and system in the body needs oxygen to function. If there is a shortage of oxygen from lung problems, digestion can suffer; muscles can cramp more easily; and fatigue, depression, and anxiety may happen. The lungs also help to rid the body of toxins, so better breathing also helps to prevent toxic overload. When a smoker gets deep breaths primarily from big drags on a cigarette, he or she does not get the full benefit of bringing in more oxygen. Deep breathing, without smoke, effectively energizes and/ or relaxes us.

Try this little experiment: pay very close attention to your experience of smoking. Before you light up in the morning, stop and take your pulse. Hold your fingers (not your thumb) over the inside of your opposite wrist, just below the thumb. For fifteen seconds, count the beats of your pulse and then multiply that number by four. Write down the number and you will have your pulse rate for one minute.

Now, light up a cigarette and take a drag. As you smoke, notice how you feel when you inhale. What sensations do you have in your chest? In your throat? Take an honest inventory of how your body feels when you breathe smoke in and out. After smoking your cigarette, take your pulse again. What is it now? Any increase gives you direct feedback on how smoking increases the workload on your heart.

Smokers typically use cigarettes to manage symptoms of stress. One of the easiest and most powerful ways to reverse stress is deep breathing. Slowing down and deepening the breath into the belly or abdomen creates a bridge from stress to relaxation. As the heart slows and blood pressure becomes normal, sleep deepens; energy, concentration, focus, and memory increase; and digestion improves.

For many people, breathing deeply and efficiently is a skill that needs to be relearned. The benefits—better relaxation and improved health—make it worthwhile. For smokers, it can also be an effective tool for delaying and stopping smoking cigarettes. Here are some exercises to explore.

Breathing Exercises

Deep abdominal breathing

1. Sit comfortably and tall in a chair with your feet flat on the floor, about shoulder width apart.

2. Start by taking in a normal breath, and then purse your lips and exhale as though you were blowing out a candle. Keep blowing until you can no longer exhale, and then allow the breath to come back in naturally. The inhalation will be deep and go to the abdomen.

3. Practice this exercise several times a day with five to ten deep breaths each time. Experiment using this practice to postpone or eliminate cigarettes.

Cleansing breath

1. Sit or stand tall. Take in as full a breath as you can, first filling the lower section of your lungs, then the middle, and then the top.

2. Puff a small breath out between pursed lips; pause and hold the breath and then puff out another breath.

3. Keep puffing and pausing until all the breath is exhaled. Repeat three or four times.

4. Relaxing sigh

5. At the same time, take in a breath and raise your shoulders up to your ears.

6. Hold the breath and shoulders for a few seconds.

7. Let your shoulders drop as you exhale with a loud sigh.

8. Repeat eight to ten times.

Deep breathing while waiting in lines

If you've caught yourself thinking that you just don't have time to practice a new skill, experiment with ways to incorporate these new habits easily into your daily activities. Standing in line for a bus or an appointment or being caught in traffic is a good time to practice a few deep breaths. Try to welcome unexpected delays as an opportunity to practice the relaxing effects of slowing down and feeling grateful for the ability to breathe fresh, smoke-free air.

4. The Psychological and Emotional Reasons for Smoking

The psychological and emotional reasons people smoke reveal that nearly all the motives to smoke are "good ones." It's just that smoking is not a healthy response to those motives. If you smoke to manage stress, be aware that much of the stress you are trying to manage is actually caused by the withdrawal symptoms that push you to reach for another smoke. Cigarettes can be used to push down difficult emotions or to deal with unpleasant situations. Discovering healthier responses to your emotional needs can enrich your life, sometimes in surprising ways.

Many smokers started smoking as teenagers, when being cool or being part of a group was a natural and important drive. Adolescence is a time of intense emotions and confusing needs. Cigarettes become a way of managing conflicting needs and muting strong feelings. Smoking can also be an initiation into appearing adult. The tobacco industry is well aware of this important adolescent drive to mimic maturity. They say that smoking is a decision that should be made by adults, not children. But what better way to convince teenagers to smoke than to tell them that choosing to smoke is a decision to be made by adults only?

If you started smoking early, what drove you to smoke as a teenager? How could you address those same drives now? As a shy teenager who was scared of being seen as uncool and unpopular,

I smoked in social settings to create the impression that I was not alone; I was just taking a cigarette break! As an adult quitting smoking, I looked at ways to cultivate an experience of belonging and to feel more comfortable in my own company. I joined a group of political activists and enjoyed meeting with other people who shared my values. There were places in my beautiful city that I'd wanted to visit, and I consciously made dates with myself to be a tourist and explore something new. Becoming aware of our motivations to smoke gives us opportunities to develop and strengthen us and to make life more interesting and rewarding.

Stress and anger management are important skills for anyone to learn, and this is no less true for smokers. I have never worked with a smoker with more pent-up stress and anger than Pete Anastole. The beginning of his journey to change was grueling. And yet, with determination, he confronted the feelings he'd been suppressing with cigarettes and transformed his vulnerability into strength. He joined a group with the shared goal of looking at angry impulses and behaviors and learned how to channel anger so he would not hurt himself or others.

When I was stopping smoking, I went to the thrift shop and loaded up on cheap, ugly plates and enjoyed the satisfaction of smashing them to bits when I felt outrage. Instead of trying to keep my "too big" emotions under control, I allowed myself to exaggerate them. When I was home alone, I would stomp around the house growling and making faces. Meditation or stress-management groups where you can also learn how to deal with difficult emotions are often available in medical settings.

The Journey of Change

A common feeling among people who have recently quit and are feeling the discomforts of adjusting to not smoking is, "How long is this going to last?" "This" refers to any of several symptoms, like irritability, sadness, and tiredness. As you can see from these interviews, the most intense discomfort after quitting can probably be measured in weeks to months. For everyone, the journey is different. However, every journey of change has general patterns that can help you when you feel lost.

Patterns of change are studied in medical settings where learning healthy behaviors is important to improved well-being. Changes tend to unfold and develop in predictable stages. In our program, we provide a map, calling it The Journey of Change.

The Journey of Change

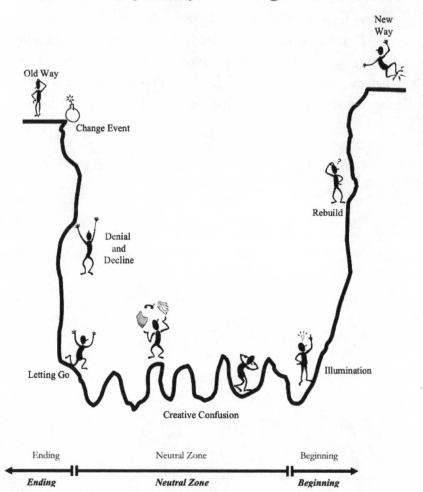

Old Way

Change Event

Denial and Decline

Letting Go

Creative Confusion

Illumination

New Way

Rebuild

Ending | Neutral Zone | Beginning

Ending | *Neutral Zone* | *Beginning*

The journey starts with ending an *Old Way* and moves to the beginning of a *New Way*. The start may be triggered by any number of events, such as leaving a home you've lived in for years, ending a relationship, or stopping smoking. These are all examples of old ways that are ending. Sometimes you can anticipate the ending as it nears. Perhaps you're aware that your relationship is not working, or maybe the company you work for has warned of layoffs. But even with the knowledge that change is approaching, when it finally happens, it can still feel like the bottom has dropped out of your life.

Moving toward a decision to stop smoking can feel the same way. You may feel alone, afraid, and even a little desperate as you set off and enter into a period of *Denial and Resistance*. Here, some or much of your energy goes into resisting change and lamenting the loss of the *Old Way*. "Why me? Why does this hurt so much? If I could just figure out how to do it right, I could get back to the Old Way." You may feel acutely aware of your attachment to the Old Way (smoking) and see more of what's wrong with the new plan and how the Old Way worked so much better. As you approach the challenge to stop smoking, you often deny that you have to change. Whatever you've been telling yourself to make smoking seem not that bad can suddenly play even louder inside your head ("I don't smoke *that* much," or "Grandpa smoked until he was ninety-three and it didn't hurt him"). Your resistance to change will eventually quiet somewhat. Maybe you get fed up with bargaining and so you let go, determined to move toward the *New Way* of a smoke-free life.

Once you really let go and stop smoking, life can get pretty confusing; nothing feels right or the same. Smoking has given structure to your daily routine for years, so when it is taken away, you are bound to feel a little lost and confused. *Creative Confusion* describes this next period. As you begin to practice living without cigarettes, you may feel exhilarated by your success and then start feeling low about how hard it is to keep from smoking. You feel fabulous and terrible, inspired and discouraged, and try a lot of new thoughts and behaviors, looking for creative solutions to becoming a non-smoker. (How do I get through the morning commute without smoking? Maybe I suck on cinnamon sticks and sing at the top of my voice. How do I manage stress without a cigarette? Maybe I remember to take five deep breaths, breathing out stress and breathing in relaxation.) Sometimes you feel like you are managing well, and at other times you feel as though something must be terribly wrong because you don't feel like yourself. Some people say they feel like a smoker who just is not smoking.

A natural part of The Journey of Change, this feeling is both confusing and creative. You feel confused and disoriented without your usual smoking, and you are creatively meeting each challenge to face life without cigarettes. It is during *Creative Confusion* that many people get discouraged and feel that it's too hard, so they turn around and go back toward the *Old Way*. All the ground you have covered is lost, and eventually you have to begin the journey all over again. I spent years in a cycle of quitting and relapsing, prolonging the very suffering I was trying to avoid.

When you enter the stage of *Creative Confusion*, you make changes in your behavior and thinking to create a life without cigarettes. In my own journey, I discovered that alcohol was a trigger for smoking and it lowered my resistance, so I chose to stay alcohol-free for a number of months. Others discover the need to adjust their caffeine intake.

After a while, and with persistence, you move through *Creative Confusion* and arrive at a place of *Illumination*. Here, there is a sense of "I see how I'm getting out of this old behavior. I still have a ways to go and more hard work to do, but I can see the direction I'm going, and I'm keeping on." The light goes on in your mind, and you begin to understand that meeting each situation as it comes will keep you moving forward to your goal of becoming a successful non-smoker.

After some time moving beyond *Illumination*, you can begin to focus on *Rebuilding* your life, continuing to learn new ways to do all the things that used to involve smoking. The low points in the journey are no longer devastating; the all or nothing feeling has pretty much gone. After I had some practice going without cigarettes and smoking no longer had the old grip on my behavior, I realized that I was safe in resuming my occasional glass of wine. Similarly, I began to reintroduce coffee into my morning routine. These are some simple examples of *Rebuilding*. Others include things like socializing in the presence of smokers and establishing healthy practices like meditation for coping with stress.

After some months of *Rebuilding*, you will arrive at the *New Way*. What stands out is a sense that being a non-smoker now feels as normal as you used to feel being a smoker. Moving through all the stages of such a journey of change typically takes about one year. Remember: this is a year when the difficult journey becomes easier and easier.

There is no way to leap over the challenges, shifts, and changes that make up The Journey of Change. The best course is to keep finding ways to push forward, knowing that with focus and persistence, you will reach the *New Smoke-Free Way*, which has become even more comfortable and rewarding than the *Old Smoker's Way*. With this map, when you find your path taking challenging turns, you can reassure yourself that it is a normal part of the journey and you can continue to push toward your goal.

In the next chapter, you will put finishing touches on your plan to stop smoking. In preparation for the final push, you have constructed a strong platform that will help you live a new life with more freedom and authenticity.

NOTES

_____

_____

_____

_____

_____

_____

_____

_____

_____

_____

_____

_____

_____

_____

_____

_____

_____

_____

_____

_____

_____

_____

CHAPTER TEN

Your Time Is Now: Gathering Resources and Successfully Stopping Smoking

Now that you are well on your way to becoming smoke-free, you are nearly ready to put cigarettes behind you. Some final preparations will set you up for success. Start by taking a look at how you organize your environment to keep smoking. If you smoke with other people, in what situations do you do that and who are those smokers? Your efforts to keep enough cigarettes on hand and to find places to smoke may be elaborate. Where do you buy your cigarettes? Do you buy packs or cartons? Do you collect matches or lighters? Understanding your patterns of keeping smoking as convenient as possible will give you the basis for rebuilding your life to keep yourself smoke-free. You could take a different route to work to avoid the store where you used to buy your cigarettes. Maybe it is important to review your social network and make new, non-smoking friends. And in preparing for your stop day, you could throw out all your cigarettes and ashtrays. Be sure to take out the trash or cover your half-smoked and leftover cigarettes with water so they can't be smoked when you get an urge.

Look at your smoking patterns. Do you smoke mostly at work or at

> "If you smoke with other people, in what situations do you do that and who are those smokers?"

"Build an awareness of your patterns so you can plan for new ones."

home? Are you alone or with other people? Do you smoke in your car or when you are bored? Build an awareness of your patterns so you can plan for new ones. With that knowledge, look at what kind of day will give you the best chances for success. Is it best to plan to quit on a day when you are busy and distracted, or would quitting on a weekend or when you have free time be better? Will you have a greater chance to get through the first days on your own or with family or friends? Will it help to be in a familiar routine or in a new one?

When you have thoroughly investigated your behavior, look at your calendar and set a stop date. Mark it on the calendar and write a personal agreement that affirms you are making this choice for yourself. Making a contract deepens your commitment to this life-supporting change. Writing it down means you'll take it more seriously. Here is a sample contract you could use or adapt for your own use. Feel free to fill it out on the next page. You can also download a printable quit plan at **www.learningtoquit.com/resources**.

Commit to Quit Agreement

On _____, I will stop using tobacco. I am agreeing to view this as a serious and important shift in my life that may lead to changes I can't predict at this point. With this commitment, I am demonstrating:

1. A sincere desire to stop

2. The motivation to make the necessary changes

3. A willingness to experience discomfort during withdrawal

I understand there will be challenging times, and I am agreeing to do my best to meet them. I will work to be kind to myself during this process and seek support when needed. By choosing to quit, I am taking a stand for my health, for the health of those around me, for the people who care about me, and, most important, for myself.

_____   _____
My Signature   *Today's Date*

Isolating and Replacing Smoking Behavior

Beginning three weeks before my own stop date, I decided to smoke in only one place. I chose my utility porch because it was the least comfortable place in my home, and it offered the fewest distractions. Whenever I wanted a cigarette, I would retreat to the back of the house and light up facing the wall of the small, cold room where my only companions were a washing machine and dryer. This practice unraveled the web of pleasures I had woven into my smoking: no more reading a book or ending a meal with a smoke; no more watching TV or visiting with a friend over cigarettes. Facing the wall in that dreary room, I found that my cigarettes began to lose their allure, and smoking began to become a boring chore. A quarter of the way through a smoke, I would get frustrated and stamp it out. By isolating my smoking behavior, I undermined associations built up over years about where and when I was accustomed to smoking. By the time my stop date arrived, I had quit smoking in so many places that my triggers were significantly reduced.

> "Facing the wall in that dreary room, I found that my cigarettes began to lose their allure, and smoking began to become a boring chore. "

I also set up a little altar—a sacred space—to honor the transition I was making and the life I was claiming. I placed a card on it with my three most important reasons for becoming smoke-free and a picture of my daughter to remind me that my efforts would have important benefits beyond my own. There was also a pretty little vase with a few fragrant flowers, so I could indulge my sense of smell as it returned after years of being suppressed by cigarettes. Over the next months, I rewarded myself for not smoking by buying whatever flowers I found most beautiful, whenever I wanted. A candle and some incense gave me healthy ways to keep matches, smoke, and flames in my life. Sitting in front of my sacred space and practicing deep-breathing exercises, I felt grateful for the gift of life. By the time my stop date arrived, I had a space where I experienced sanctuary and pleasure, a place where I could continue to nurture the new identity I was growing: being a non-smoker!

If you were to limit yourself to one place to smoke, where would that be? If you have been smoking inside your home, you might want to make your place somewhere outside. That way, once you have reached your stop date, you will already have built up an association of being smoke-free at home. By stopping smoking inside, you will give yourself the added satisfaction of knowing that you are protecting your loved ones from the dangers of second- and third-hand smoke.

Some smokers write a farewell letter to their cigarettes. You could begin your letter by thanking cigarettes for all they have given you in your life and then explain why you have decided it is time to say goodbye. Take a moment to jot down a few thoughts about what might go into your own goodbye letter.

Making a Quit Plan

Becoming a successful non-smoker is about strategy, not willpower. A detailed and well-thought-out quit plan creates the best odds for success. Being prepared means that when you are faced with urges in difficult situations, you will be ready to deal with them. In the journey to stopping smoking, think in terms of three phases: getting ready, scheduling your actual stop date, and staying on course. Write out your plan, describing the actions you will take, including a Plan B in case Plan A needs backup. You can use the quit plan template on the next page to guide you.

My Quit Plan

Phase	Actions I will take	Plan B *(if needed)*
Getting Ready Adjust Environment Nicotine Replacement Medications Language Support Systems Denial Story Other		*Important:* If you don't outline a Plan B and you begin to struggle, your Plan B will automatically be a cigarette.
My Stop Date General Approach Ceremony Medications Urge Response Special Plans Friends and Family Other		
Staying on Course Urge Response Withdrawal Coping Danger-Zone Strategy Medication Compliance Language Courage Support Systems Relapse Prevention Celebration Rewards Other		

Download a printable quit plan at **www.learningtoquit.com/resources**.

When you get ready, think about how to adjust your environment. Include things like clearing out ashtrays and lighters, putting up encouraging signs, and letting friends and family know your home is going to be smoke-free. Make decisions about any medications (NRT, Zyban, Chantix) you want to use and arrange to purchase them and/or obtain prescriptions from your doctor. Think about the language you want to use in talking with yourself, and develop a mantra to keep you focused on your goal. As I have shared, mine was *I am smoke free, fearless, and proud.* How will you get support, and who will be your support system? What is your denial story, and how can you fight it so it doesn't have the power to lure you back to smoking?

What will be your approach on the day you quit? Do you want to create a ceremony to mark the transition into your new way of life? Will you write a farewell letter to cigarettes, thanking them for all they have provided and describing why you have chosen to say goodbye? What skills and tools will you use to meet urges? Perhaps you will use a short-acting nicotine replacement therapy (NRT) medication for sudden strong urges. Deep breathing can calm urges. It can also be helpful to make special plans for the first few smoke-free days. What about spending time where you *can't* smoke: in the movies; at the library; or in a mosque, synagogue, or church? Would you find it supportive to spend time with friends or family, or would you rather be alone? To stay on course, you will need a variety of choices to manage urges. One couple I know chose to stop smoking together on a weekend. They decided to minimize stress, sleeping in late and having a variety of fun activities to keep themselves busy and distracted. They also agreed to an emotional buffer zone. That way, if one of them was feeling irritable or short-tempered, they would acknowledge their discomfort and ask for a time-out.

Tips for the Day You Quit

It bears repeating that preparation is key to success; strategy trumps willpower. By your stop date, you will have prepared yourself, your environment, and your support network. You will have cleared out all your cigarettes, being sure to check pockets, handbags, the spaces between your couch cushions, and under car seats. You'll have thrown away all your ashtrays or transformed any that have special meaning into containers for special items. You'll have prepared for this day by making plans for what you will do and how you will reward yourself.

Going to work, select a different route. Make plans for how you will take breaks that do not involve smoking. Assess routines for ways you can change those breaks to support smoke-free behaviors. In the morning, sit somewhere other than in your favorite smoking chair, and maybe start the day with tea instead of coffee. Keep yourself busy, especially your hands. Be sure to build physical exercise into your daily regimen. A brisk walk will help alleviate withdrawal symptoms, and deep breathing will clear out your lungs more quickly. Get adequate rest, and if you find yourself feeling sleepy with withdrawal symptoms, take naps and go to bed earlier.

People have different ways of meeting the sometimes-grueling urges that can arise, particularly in the first week or two of letting go of smoking. Some go day by day, others moment by moment or breath by breath. Remember, you only have to take on one urge at a time. No one ever dies from resisting an urge to smoke, and even if you do not do anything about it, an urge passes in just a few minutes. You can help yourself by reviewing your "want to" list and by celebrating and rewarding yourself for your efforts. Keep saying your mantra, and even if you think "I can have just one puff," remember not to believe it. Just because you thought it does not mean you have to have the cigarette.

Get a **Tips for the Day You Quit** checklist at
www.learningtoquit.com/resources.

Using the Five D's to Deal with Urges

Urges to smoke are normal and do not mean anything is wrong. Over the years, you have trained your brain to look forward to smoking in many situations, and now you are choosing to end that behavior pattern. Initially, your body is going to feel that what is happening is unnatural. But each urge and each withdrawal symptom is actually part of the process your body goes through as it heals from a powerful addiction.

Many former smokers discovered that stopping was not as hard as they expected, and they wished they had done it sooner. For most smokers, stopping is not easy, and it is critical to have a plan, especially for how to get through the early stages. A good strategy is to rely on the Five Ds, which are simple, free, and almost always available:

1. **Drink water.** Drinking water gives your hands and mouth something to do, helps to flush toxins, and is a healthy alternative to lighting up. Linda McNicoll (Chapter Five) found this to be a good strategy for helping to control urges to overeat. Whenever she felt anxious or felt the urge to smoke, she'd drink from the water bottle she kept nearby at all times.

2. **Delay the craving** is a very adaptable *D*. "If I still feel this way tomorrow, I will have a cigarette." Then, when tomorrow comes, "If I still feel this way tomorrow …." In this way, smoking keeps getting put off. Cecilia Brunazzi (Page One) adapted this coping mechanism to minutes or hours instead of a whole day. There is no need to scare yourself with thoughts like, "Oh dear, I can never have another cigarette again, ever." Such thoughts can create the anxiety that triggers smoking. All that is necessary is to remind yourself that in this moment you will be smoke-free. That way, moment by moment, you are building your new identity and reality as a non-smoker.

3. **Do something else.** If you are hit with an urge to smoke, no matter what you happen to be doing at that moment, make a shift. If you are reading in the living room, go to the kitchen and make a pot of tea. If you are at the computer, go outside and take a brisk walk. Changing what you are doing can do wonders for changing what you are thinking and feeling.

4. **Deep breathe.** Breathing deeply into the abdomen is a powerful, quick, and easy way to induce relaxation. Remember Clarence Brown's assertion that deep abdominal breathing was what helped him more than anything to become and stay smoke-free? Taking a deep breath brings more oxygen and relaxation into your body. Breathing deeply helps you get through urges more quickly and with less discomfort.

5. **Discuss with a friend.** If you are having a rough time navigating your new smoke-free life, call someone who will understand and support you. This may be someone who is a former smoker and can relate to your experience. Or perhaps it's someone who is working to make changes in his or her own life, possibly with diet or exercise, and in solidarity can help cheer you on your way. Joyce Lavey (Chapter Five) kept a list of phone numbers of people who were willing to be called, and when she was feeling threatened by overwhelming urges, she'd call an understanding and supportive friend for reinforcement. Who would your person be?

Download a printable "5 D's" PDF at **www.learningtoquit.com/resources**.

Rewards and Celebrations

An important part of any big behavioral change is remembering to give yourself credit for your hard work. Sometimes people go back to smoking by undervaluing their accomplishment with thoughts like, "It wasn't that hard to quit. I can have just one." Keep in mind that if you could have just one, then your last one would've been the *last one*. To protect yourself against relapse, practice rewarding and celebrating your success frequently. Especially in the initial stages of cessation, you can feel excited and exhilarated by your accomplishments. By the third or fourth week, the excitement may have waned and perhaps your support network has lost sight of the importance of what you're doing. Celebrating and rewarding your smoke-free choices helps to reprogram your mind with new thoughts and beliefs about what is normal. Use any excuse to reward yourself: if you avoid a situation where you know you'd like to smoke, if you see cigarettes and don't pick one up, if you visit your in-laws and don't take a smoke break, if you decide not to smoke after an argument, or if you decide not to bum a cigarette from a coworker. In any of these situations, you could reward yourself in many different ways: get a massage, go to a movie, put a gold star on your calendar, go out to dinner with a friend, or simply pat yourself on the back. You might use the money you would have spent on cigarettes to buy yourself something you want but wouldn't have bought otherwise.

> "Use any excuse to reward yourself."

Every time you take a puff of a cigarette, no matter what else is happening, the quick burst of nicotine to the brain stimulates a release of dopamine, the chemical that gives you the sensations of pleasure and reward. In fact, *every* pleasurable experience requires the release of dopamine to be felt at all. And one of the reasons you got hooked on smoking is because of the dopamine that was released. You can be very ill with a cold or the flu, for example, and smoke a cigarette, coughing and gasping for breath. But because taking those puffs releases dopamine, you experience the cigarette as rewarding. When you are learning to become a non-smoker, choosing things to give yourself a feeling of reward is beneficial to reclaiming the natural release of dopamine.

Some smokers in this book rewarded themselves in big ways with long-term savings. Pete Anastole, who had been a heavy smoker, used the money he saved to buy a truck. Sandy had little to no spending money and used her cigarette savings to buy books that provided her with an escape from thinking about smoking.

As you continue to be smoke-free, you deserve to feel proud, confident, and strong. Some people don't find it easy to reward themselves and may even have a hard time thinking of what might feel rewarding. Remember, every cigarette you used to smoke gave you the experience of reward. So finding ways to acknowledge your hard work with healthy rewards is an important part of healing. What might be some short-term and some long-term rewards for you? Take a few minutes now to write down a list of rewards you could enjoy. You deserve them.

Relapse Prevention

As you log more time and become a non-smoker, you are likely to encounter challenges and setbacks. If you find yourself slipping or taking a detour, get back on the right road as soon as possible. Not all detours are the same. and knowing the differences can be helpful. Relapse has three levels: a lapse, a relapse, and a collapse.

With a *lapse*, you decide to smoke one or a few cigarettes, and then within a very short time, you return to being smoke-free. A lapse can last from a few minutes up to a day or two.

In a true *relapse*, you return to square one. You decide to smoke, and within a short time, you are back to smoking the same amount as before your quit date. Once you've relapsed, you need to recommit and start again.

> "A lapse can last from a few minutes up to a day or two."

A *collapse* is to be avoided at all costs. In a collapse, you not only decide to smoke and quickly return to your pre-quit level of smoking, but you also lose faith in yourself. You use the detour as proof that you may never be able to become smoke-free. By thinking, "I can't do this; I am doomed to be a smoker for the rest of my life," you are worse off than you were before you attempted to stop. This is a state of mind only you can decide to avoid.

> "Once you've relapsed, you need to recommit and start again."

A relapse begins before you actually pick up the cigarette. The mind, in its effort to pull you back into familiar behaviors, will look for ways to set the stage for relapse. The relapse process is an energetic buildup leading back to smoking. Paying attention to your thoughts will help prevent a relapse by alerting you to interrupt this energetic buildup. You can be aware of the mental progression to relapse by monitoring your thoughts and stopping problems before they have a chance to develop.

Let's look at this relapse progression in more detail.

1. The first step on the road comes with considering even a small possibility that you will smoke again sometime in the future.

2. Once you accept the idea that such a possibility exists, your mind begins to search for conditions that would provide permission to smoke. Some people think, "I'll be okay as long as I don't have too much stress." Now the mind knows what conditions would make it okay to smoke: stress. It doesn't even have to be a particularly challenging stressor—it could be something as simple as your partner neglecting to take out the trash. "How could he *do* that? Doesn't he know I'm trying to stop smoking? That's so inconsiderate. He knows enough to take out the trash, so he's just being thoughtless and insensitive. I'll just have to smoke."

3. If you don't get derailed right away, once you've accepted the possibility that you'll smoke again, your mind begins to anticipate, maybe even fantasize about this possible smoking experience.

4. Left ignored, anticipation grows into actual craving, which keeps building until it's intolerable. You rethink how small that initial possibility really is. The conditions under which you smoke become less vague and now include more likely situations. You've set the stage for clear permission to smoke, and it's just a matter of time before you do it.

In summary, the road to relapse begins with a small possibility leading to craving, which leads to clear permission, and then smoking. Being familiar with these mental patterns can give you a jump on disrupting this progression before it ends with a cigarette.

Looking at the structure of relapse reveals that smoking tobacco causes changes in the brain. Nicotine in cigarette smoke is carried rapidly to the brain (within five heartbeats), where it attaches to receptors. Receptors in the brain are like the lock to your front door. They are restricted in what they will recognize and in what can attach to them. Once the receptors become accustomed to a certain level of nicotine, you will experience withdrawal symptoms when they don't get their usual dose. When you stop smoking, over time the number of these receptors begins to return to normal. However, once receptors are exposed and dependent on nicotine, they maintain a memory of your nicotine requirements as a smoker. That is why when a former smoker has even a puff of a cigarette, even years after quitting, the receptors begin wanting more nicotine, and the former smoker has to struggle against urges which, if ignored, take them back to their old daily intake.

As I am writing this, I am 66 years old and have not smoked in more than thirty years. If I had *never* smoked and decided to try it at my age, the cigarette would taste nasty and harsh and make me cough and feel dizzy and nauseated. Nothing about the experience would tempt me to continue to smoke more. However, I *do* have a history of tobacco dependence. So if I had even a single puff of a cigarette today, even with the predictable symptoms of coughing and nausea, my receptors would immediately remember former smoking reward experiences and begin wanting more nicotine. Like the people I've worked with who relapsed decades after quitting, I could soon return to my earlier levels of smoking. You can use this information to empower yourself to avoid falling back into dependency.

Whenever you find yourself having a thought such as, "It won't hurt to have just one," remind yourself that that's a lie. All it would take to reawaken the desire to smoke nicotine is a minimal exposure, and then you would be faced with struggling to quit cigarettes all over again.

One Final Exercise

Before you move on to the conclusion of this chapter, here is one last exercise to help focus and direct whatever skills are most powerful for you. With a fresh piece of paper, sit down and write yourself a letter. You can use the blank pages at the end of this chapter. Date your letter six months from now, and begin by saying, "I am a successful non-smoker." Go on to describe in detail the challenges you faced and the skills you used to overcome them. Describe your insights and accomplishments as though they are in the past and fully achieved. Describe specific goals you reached.

> Sit down and write yourself a letter. You can use the blank pages at the end of this chapter. Date your letter six months from now. Write: "I am a successful non-smoker." Go on to describe in detail the challenges you faced and the skills you used to overcome them.

Be sure to include how you are feeling being smoke-free. How have your feelings about yourself changed? What are you feeling physically? What are some of the things you have discovered about yourself in the process of becoming a non-smoker? Be as descriptive and as detailed in your letter as you can. This is a letter at the beginning of your new life, free of smoking. Writing it out in full detail will give you both the plan for what that new life will look and feel like, and a descriptive road map to get you to your goal.

Benefits of Quitting

One of the exciting benefits of becoming smoke-free is a whole new relationship with your body and your health. You will have the pleasure of knowing you are taking care of yourself and your future. Using some of the awareness practices discussed here, you will have greater access to your feelings and your true self without the suppressing effects of smoking.

The best news about becoming smoke-free is that it really makes a difference. Our bodies have an amazing capacity for healing. No matter when you stop smoking, your health can improve. Here are just some of the powerful benefits that will be yours as you recover from tobacco dependence.

Within 20 minutes of your last cigarette:

- You stop polluting the air with dangerous second-hand smoke

- Blood pressure drops to normal

- Pulse rate drops to normal

- Temperature of hands and feet increases to normal

24 hours:

- Chance of heart attack decreases

48 hours:

- Carbon monoxide level in blood returns to normal

- Oxygen level in blood increases to normal

- Nerve endings adjust to the absence of nicotine

- Ability to smell and taste is enhanced

72 hours:

- Bronchial tubes relax, making breathing easier

- Lung capacity increases

Two weeks to three months:

- Circulation improves

- Walking becomes easier

One to nine months:

- Coughing, sinus congestion, fatigue, and shortness of breath decrease

- Cilia regrow in lungs, increasing the ability to clean the lungs and reduce infection

- The body's overall energy level increases

One year:

- Heart-disease death rate is halfway back to that of a nonsmoker

Five years:

- Heart-disease death rate drops to the rate of non-smokers
- Lung cancer death rate decreases halfway back to that of non-smokers

Ten years:

- Lung cancer death rate drops almost to the rate for non-smokers
- Precancerous cells are replaced
- Incidence of other cancers, such as mouth, larynx, esophagus, bladder, kidney, and pancreas decreases
- Fifteen years:
- Risk of lung cancer is reduced to close to that observed in non-smokers
- Risk of coronary artery disease falls to the same as someone who has never smoked
- If you have quit smoking before the age of fifty, you have halved the risk of dying in the next fifteen years compared with continuing smokers

This timetable of recovery shows many of the tremendous benefits of stopping smoking. It reminds me of an evening when my three-year-old grandson, who is an authority on dinosaurs, shared his understanding of their survival and transformation. He explained that the dinosaurs had "survolved" into some of the birds we see today. I have loved that word since I first heard him say it, and I think it beautifully captures the process of becoming smoke-free. You will survive the challenges of the process of stopping smoking, and by doing so, you will evolve into greater health and freedom. May you "survolve" into a healthy, happy non-smoker.

NOTES

_____

_____

_____

_____

_____

_____

_____

_____

_____

_____

_____

_____

_____

_____

_____

_____

_____

_____

_____

_____

NOTES

NOTES

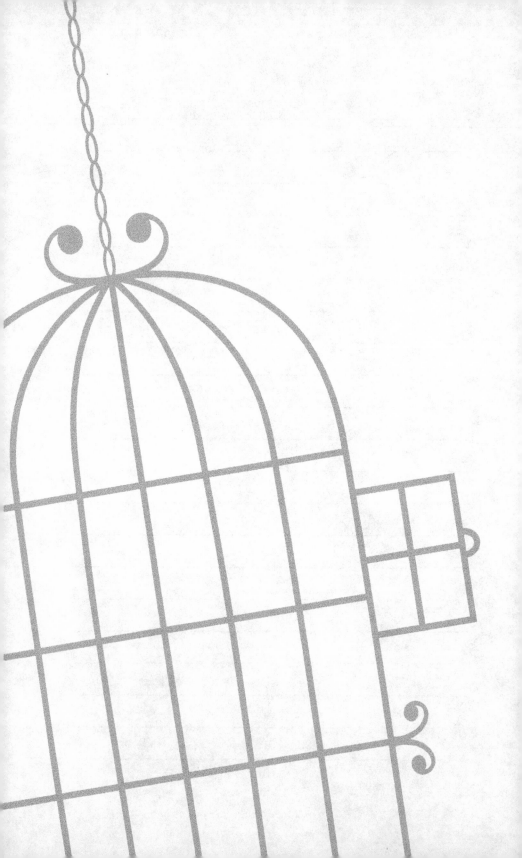

PART TWO

Information That Can Support Your Quit Plan

CHAPTER ELEVEN
Tobacco and Lung Disease

Adapt what is useful, reject what is useless, and add what is specifically your own. **Bruce Lee**

Tar—it's in every cigarette you smoke and directly causes many of the diseases that you want to avoid. Tar droplets in smoke are inhaled into your mouth, throat, and lungs, and nicotine hitches a ride on this tar. Not only does tar contain carcinogens, which are cancer-causing chemicals, it also contains thousands of other chemicals. Tar is the main vehicle to drive nicotine to your lungs where nicotine is rapidly absorbed in seconds and reaches your brain after a few heartbeats.

Your lungs were never designed for repeated smoke exposure. They respond by continually working to repair the damage that occurs from smoke. This chapter will describe the way cigarette smoking can cause lung disease, but there are many other diseases that smoking worsens or increases the risk of their development. These can include Alzheimer's disease, rheumatoid arthritis, erectile dysfunction, cataracts, age-related macular degeneration, and several others.

Lung disease is one of the most common problems caused by cigarette smoking. Chapter Eleven will describe some of the basic information you need to know about emphysema and chronic bronchitis (which, together, form Chronic Obstructive Pulmonary Disease (COPD). In addition, it covers the effect of carbon monoxide, and symptoms such as shortness of breath and coughs. Lung cancer is discussed in a Chapter Thirteen.

Normal Lung Function

Your lungs have roughly the surface area of a tennis court, all packed into your chest cavity (Figure 1). This amazing design is made possible by millions of tiny air sacs attached to tubes that get smaller and smaller the farther away they are from your large windpipe (the trachea).

- Your lungs resemble an upside-down tree, with the windpipe acting as the trunk.
- Just as a tree develops a large surface area by growing thousands of leaves, we humans have developed a huge surface area in our lungs, with millions of air sacs.
- Our large airways are hollow branches that get smaller until finally they end with microscopic air sacs called alveoli.
- These air sacs are surrounded by capillaries, the smallest blood vessels in the body.

As air is pulled into the lungs, it inflates the alveoli, allowing for the normal movement of oxygen from the air into the blood vessels that surround these air sacs. At the same time as this is happening, the cells in our body produce carbon dioxide as a waste product. It's transported in the bloodstream to the lungs and gets released into the air sacs and is breathed out when you exhale. Your lungs allow this constant exchange of oxygen in and carbon dioxide out with every breath you take.

As you read this, take a deep, deep breath in and hold it. Now let that air out—it rushes out easily, because your lung tissue is firm like a sponge and the air tubes are open. Oxygen in the air is critical to the function of every cell in your body—without it, you'd die in minutes.

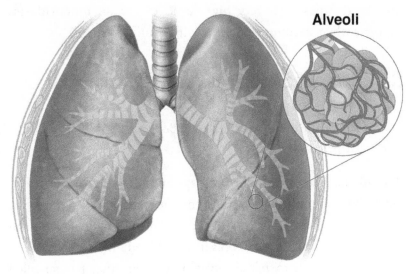

Alveoli

Figure 1: Trachea, lungs, and main airways.

What happens when you smoke?

Oxygen transport from the air into your body is going on every second of every day. This changes if you're a smoker, because lighting a cigarette generates smoke and carbon monoxide which is breathed deeply into your lungs.

- Anything that burns creates carbon monoxide, an odorless, tasteless, and colorless gas.
- With carbon monoxide around, the hemoglobin (which transports oxygen) in your red blood cells can't bind to oxygen properly to transport and release it in the tissues.
- The amount of oxygen available to the smoker has been lowered. You may feel short of breath when exercising with an elevated carbon monoxide level.

Smokers typically have higher levels of carbon monoxide than non-smokers. Elevated carbon monoxide can be detected by a carbon monoxide monitor (which may be available at your local medical center if you want to take an easy breathing test). Carbon monoxide poisoning can occur when people are in an enclosed space and exposed to very high levels of carbon monoxide (as happens when sleeping in a house with a faulty furnace).

The Effects of Smoking on Lung Function

Chronic Obstructive Pulmonary Disease—Emphysema and Chronic Bronchitis

Beyond the role of transporting oxygen and carbon dioxide, our lungs constantly interact with the environment by processing dust, bacteria and viruses that we breathe in day and night. If a foreign material is inhaled, immune cells in your blood find it and attack it.

In Figure 2, there's an alveolus (air sac) that has tar-filled immune cells in it. These scavenger cells are found in the lungs of regular smokers, and they do the work of clearing tar deposited in the airways and air sacs of the lungs every day. This is your immune system's response to a foreign material in an otherwise sterile environment, and once the immune cell surrounds the tar, it breaks it down in an effort to destroy it. This inflammation can cause widespread damage to the airways in the form of chronic bronchitis and damage to the airspaces in the form of emphysema.

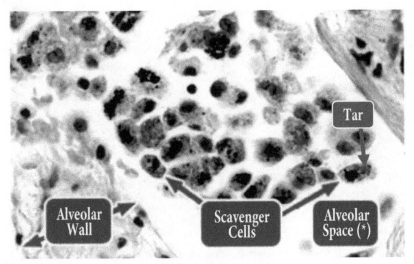

Figure 2: Scavenger cells (macrophages) filled with tar in your air sacs.
Source: www.medicine.com

Cigarette smoking is the leading cause of Chronic Obstructive Pulmonary Disease (COPD). Common symptoms of COPD are coughing, wheezing, and a reduced ability to force air out of your lungs. The two main forms of COPD are **chronic bronchitis** and **emphysema**.

Bronchitis is inflammation in the medium-sized air passages in your lungs.

- Acute bronchitis causes coughing and shortness of breath and is often associated with infections from bacteria or viruses.

- Chronic bronchitis is due in large part to cigarette smoking and is defined as a daily cough that produces mucus every day for at least three continuous months for two years in a row.

In both cases, the bronchi become inflamed and narrowed, and mucus increases tremendously from the inflamed cells in your airways. Narrowed air passages can result in the feeling of tightness in your chest, shortness of breath, cough, and/or wheezing. Figure 3 shows you a normal airway and an airway with chronic bronchitis.

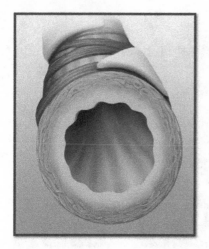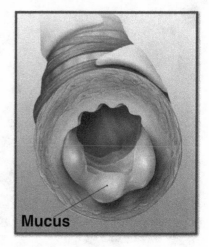

Mucus

Figure 3: Normal bronchi without inflammation and with chronic bronchitis.

Emphysema is different from chronic bronchitis, and smokers are at significant risk of developing emphysema as Bill Andrews did, as described in Chapter Three. Emphysema is caused by the constant destruction of normal lung tissue and is a leading cause of chronic illness in smokers.

As lung tissue is destroyed, the air sacs and small airways become moth-eaten in appearance. Normally strong and spongy lung tissue becomes thin (Figure 4). Delicate walls between the air sacs are destroyed. The overall lung surface area becomes gradually and permanently reduced. Imagine a healthy tree gradually stripped of its leaves—the same loss of surface area occurs as alveoli are destroyed. We don't have the ability to significantly reverse this process. Some people develop large air pockets in their lungs, and these air pockets can push on normal lung tissue, making this situation even worse.

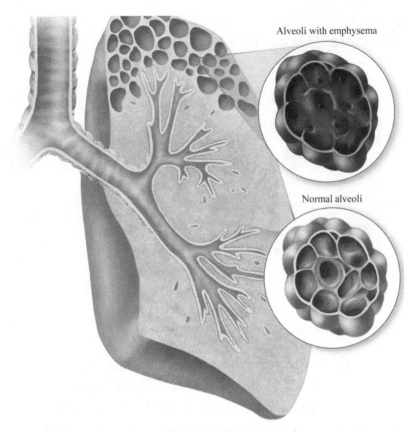

Alveoli with emphysema

Normal alveoli

Figure 4: Normal air sacs (alveoli) and alveoli with emphysema.

More than 80 percent of cases of emphysema are caused by smoking, making them completely preventable. If patients develop severe disease, they may be hospitalized for even minor lung infections, and need steroids like prednisone to reduce inflammation, antibiotics to treat infection, and oxygen—they might even have to be placed on life support in the intensive care unit (as Clarence Brown was, as described in Chapter Eight).

Everyone loses some degree of lung function as they get older, but the loss is relatively minor and largely unnoticed. Figure 5 shows the normal and expected loss of the ability to breathe out forcefully in one second plotted against age. People who never smoked have an expected mild decline, but smokers may have a much more rapid decline that can worsen with age and lead to serious disability unless smoke exposure is stopped. This rapid decline can be greatly slowed if a smoker with COPD quits successfully.

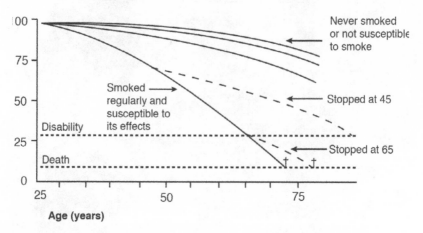

Figure 5: Normal decline of lung function with age and rapid decline with smoking.
Data from Fletcher and Peto, 1977.

Changes in lung function can be easily measured by pulmonary function tests. A technician enters your basic information, like age, weight, and height, and then has you breathe in and out through a tube you place in your mouth and seal with your lips. Lung function tests are simple and painless and can be done in a routine office visit.

We take our lung function for granted until we have a significant problem, and then we may try to compensate by being less active to reduce the symptoms. This kind of behavior change can start a slow, worsening cycle of decline in your health, and it increases your risk for all sorts of complications like heart failure, pneumonia, and other conditions. Once lung destruction is advanced, inhaled medications that keep the airways open are less effective over time, as was the case with Bill Andrews, as described in Chapter Three.

The Meaning of Shortness of Breath

During your normal activities, your body can efficiently transport oxygen from your lungs to your tissues, and you don't feel the sensation that you need more air. If this process is inefficient or abnormal, sensors in the brain and lungs will generate signals that you should breathe more, and you'll experience the sensation of breathlessness. If you're healthy and in good physical shape and are asked to walk up two flights of stairs quickly, after fifteen to twenty steps you'll begin to notice you're breathing harder and feeling slightly short of breath. You might notice mild and short-lived tiredness in your legs, but this and the shortness of breath will pass in seconds once you stop. This happens because your muscles use up oxygen faster than it can be supplied. Your brain sends the signal to breathe faster and deeper, and you do, until you generate a supply of oxygen that catches up with the demand and the shortness of breath goes away.

If you have shortness of breath at rest or with even mild exercise, such as a walk across a room, this is abnormal and needs to be evaluated. There are several potential explanations for this shortness of breath. These may include a primary lung problem (emphysema) or potentially a heart problem. Perhaps, as a smoker, your carbon monoxide level is elevated, and even a small amount of exercise triggers the shortness of breath. This is a potentially serious symptom that needs medical attention.

If you have any symptoms at all, you should have your lungs tested with simple breathing tests that can be arranged through your regular doctor.

The Significance of a Cough

Coughing is triggered by inflammation in the air passages. It is meant to expel foreign bodies or mucus during an infection. In general, your lungs are relatively insensitive to minor changes. For this reason, minor alterations in your airways might go unnoticed. Cough receptors at major branch points in your airways are more sensitive than the rest of your lung tissue. Since your lungs are generally not very sensitive, a slow-growing tumor could develop entirely without symptoms until it becomes large enough to irritate a sensitive area of your airways or the lining around the lungs or your chest wall.

Persistent cough—coughing repeatedly through the day or at night—is abnormal. Chronic bronchitis can cause a chronic cough. Asthma, infections, or tumors also can cause this cough. If you're experiencing frequent coughing, and especially if you are coughing up blood or have chest discomfort, see a health care provider right away.

The Benefits of Quitting

When you stop smoking, your lung health may be able to return to the near normal rate of slow decline expected with age (Figure 5). While approximately 20 percent to 25 percent of smokers are susceptible to COPD, it's possible to have mild disease in your thirties and without feeling any symptoms. Quitting can stop the rapid decline in lung function seen in some smokers, thereby preventing a future life of minimal activity and possible oxygen-tank use.

Once you stop smoking, carbon monoxide is cleared from your lungs and body over days. This difference alone may significantly reduce any shortness of breath you experience. Try to measure how far you can normally walk before you notice a slight shortness of breath. Is it one block or five? Set a baseline for yourself, and then follow it during the course of quitting. If you notice shortness of breath before you quit, you might see an improvement within the first few days.

As for cough, it's known that smoking interferes with the normal clearance of mucus from your airways. When some smokers quit, they notice an increased cough for several days. This is actually a good sign. Your body is working to clear out tar and mucus. Drinking plenty of water should help. Imagine your thickened airways generating less mucus and returning to normal over time. Imagine those scavenger immune cells finally able to complete their task of clearing tar from the airways. A chronic bronchitis–associated cough is significantly improved with smoking cessation, and you lower the chance of having acute bronchitis attacks after you quit.

What You Need to Know

- Lung health is directly related to quality of life. How well we're able to breathe affects how we live, sleep, and function and has a major impact on our state of mind.
- Smoking speeds up aging of the lungs and can cause chronic bronchitis and emphysema.
- Symptoms of shortness of breath or chronic cough should be evaluated. Ask your doctor for a breathing test to check your lung function.
- Symptoms of shortness of breath, muscle fatigue, and cough can improve after stopping smoking.
- Stopping smoking leads to improved lung function and a slowing of the aging process.
- No matter how we might have damaged our health by smoking, stopping can make a difference.

CHAPTER TWELVE

Smoking and Cardiovascular Health

The most difficult thing is the decision to act; the rest is merely tenacity. **Amelia Earhart**

Most people are aware of the link between smoking and the risk of a heart attack or stroke, but the knowledge often ends there. How does smoking increase these risks? You might not know how smoking increases the risk of heart attack or stroke or peripheral vascular disease. Or how this risk differs from one person to the next. One of the most important facts is that a heart attack or stroke can happen quickly and without warning. The stories of Dr. Ernie Ring in Chapter Two and R.E.C. in Chapter Three are classic examples of the consequence of suddenly changing the blood flow to the heart.

According to the Centers for Disease Control, every year in the United States, approximately 735,000 people have heart attacks, and 800,000 people experience strokes. Smoking can contribute to the risk of

"The most common risk factors for a heart attack are cigarette smoking, diabetes, high blood pressure, family history of a heart attack, and high cholesterol."

sudden death, which is typically due to a heart attack, an abnormal heart rhythm, or a large blood clot in the lung circulation. The most common risk factors for a heart attack are cigarette smoking, diabetes, high blood pressure, family history of a heart attack, and high cholesterol. The risks of these events are much higher in smokers, making cigarette smoking the most significant cause of preventable heart disease.

"If blood flow to your heart or brain is stopped due to a heart attack or stroke, you could pass out in seconds and be dead in minutes."

Every cell and tissue in your body needs two basic elements to survive: oxygen and a sugar molecule called glucose. Oxygen comes from the air you breathe, and glucose comes from the breakdown of foods in your digestive system. Oxygen and glucose in blood are pumped through your arteries by the heart.

If blood flow to your heart or brain is stopped due to a heart attack or stroke, you could pass out in seconds and be dead in minutes, in part because the heart and brain have the highest needs for oxygen and glucose in the body.

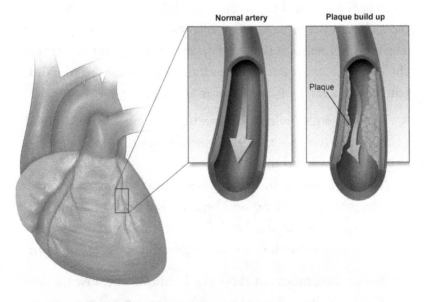

Figure 6. The heart, a coronary artery, and plaque build-up.

Do you remember the first cigarette you had? Nicotine was absorbed into your bloodstream and crossed quickly into your brain. Tar and thousands of chemicals were absorbed and sent throughout your body. Carbon monoxide from the cigarette smoke was absorbed into your bloodstream and reduced the delivery of oxygen to your tissues (more on this in Chapter Twelve). Nicotine, in the high concentrations that spike when you smoke a cigarette, causes your body to release adrenaline and this increases your heart rate and blood pressure, effectively increasing the work of your heart.

Putting your blood vessels through this assault multiple times every day, day after day, has a major impact on your heart and circulatory health. Humans aren't designed to handle this constant stress without eventually suffering the consequences. When we're young, we're able to recover from this harm far better than when we're older, and many of the wide-ranging effects of smoking are cumulative. In fact, recent studies suggest that if you successfully quit smoking by the age of thirty, your life expectancy could be close to normal. And quitting smoking at any age has immediate benefits.

Smoking can cause a change in the normal processing of lipids or fats in your body, including triglycerides. Triglycerides are the main form of fat in your fat cells and in your circulating blood. Triglyceride levels are increased from smoking, and HDL (good cholesterol) is decreased. **These changes increase the likelihood you'll form a fatty plaque in your arteries.**

- As this plaque builds up, it can begin to block normal blood flow, and this blockage is worsened when the blood vessel constricts around the plaque.
- The plaque found in smokers is also unstable compared to what happens with nonsmokers and is prone to rupture, causing a clot that can break free and get carried downstream and reduce blood flow to vital organs like the heart or brain.

- The clotting process is abnormal in smokers because the sticky platelets that are floating in the bloodstream can form clots after a local plaque rupture.

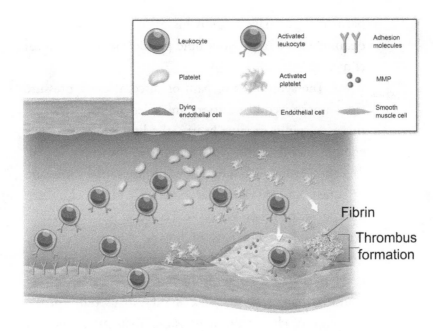

Figure 7: Inflammatory effects of smoking on plaque formation.

So, as in Figure 6 and 7, imagine a narrowed artery that gets squeezed further during smoking. As a plaque ruptures, a blood clot can block the arteries of the heart or brain and cause a sudden heart attack or stroke in the area the clogged artery normally supplies. This increased potential for plaque formation, rupture, and clotting is why patients with heart attacks or strokes are routinely placed on blood thinners like aspirin and other drugs.

The silent process of plaque build-up occurs over many years, and you don't feel it. It's a gradual process that becomes riskier as you move into your forties and fifties. Other factors like diabetes or hypertension or high cholesterol speed up this process. A family history of heart attack, stroke, or sudden death can definitely identify you as being at higher risk of coronary artery disease. This may suggest an inherited mutation in the genes that control lipid and cholesterol production and

"If you have a family history of heart disease, you definitely need to get your lipid profile checked at a local clinic."

balance. If you have a family history of heart disease, you definitely need to get your lipid profile checked at a local clinic.

The symptoms of pain or discomfort or pressure from a narrowed heart artery are called angina. Think of this as a cramp in your heart—the heart doesn't receive enough blood supply and sends you a warning signal. The chest pain is often described as heavy, like a pressure or squeezing sensation that can travel to the shoulder, neck, arm, or other locations. People might have vague symptoms like shortness of breath, nausea, vomiting, sweating, dizziness, or others. Women might experience less pain than men, and for them, coronary artery disease could be harder to diagnose if they focus only on the symptom of chest pain or pressure. There are no perfect diagnostic symptoms, so the best approach is to talk to a doctor and determine if some simple tests can help determine if you have tobacco-related cardiovascular disease.

> "Smoking is a risk factor for the development of a heart attack or stroke, even if you don't have other risks."

There are times when heart attacks or strokes can occur in smokers of an even younger age. Women who smoke and use birth control pills or contraceptive rings are at a significantly higher risk of a heart attack or leg clots. People with autoimmune diseases including rheumatoid arthritis, lupus, and vasculitis are more prone to these events. Remember that smoking is a risk factor for the development of a heart attack or stroke, even if you don't have other risks.

The best news is that *your heart and circulatory health improves quickly when you stop smoking.* The carbon monoxide in your bloodstream begins to decrease. People often say that breathing is easier within days of quitting. Over the course of months, the normal balance of fat metabolism, platelet stickiness, and blood-vessel contraction can return. Focusing on a healthy diet and gradually increasing your exercise, simply by walking, will strengthen the major benefits of quitting.

Many smokers fear that they will gain weight after quitting. This can be five to ten pounds (4–5 kg) on average, unless you have a plan. It is far less risky to gain a little weight compared to continued smoking. In the best case, you will quit smoking and, in the process, increase your exercise as part of your plan—two extraordinary benefits to your heart health as you are learning to quit.

What You Need to Know

- Smoking alters the processing of lipids (fat) in your body. This can increase plaque formation in your arteries, including the arteries in your heart.
- Smoking increases clotting of blood around a plaque.
- If you develop plaques in your arteries, smoking can increase the likelihood of plaque rupture.
- Nicotine increases constriction of blood vessels.
- Smoking causes increased heart rate and blood pressure. This increases the work of your heart.
- Carbon monoxide from smoking reduces oxygen delivery to all your organs, including your heart.
- Many of these negative effects of smoking are reversed in the first year after quitting.

CHAPTER THIRTEEN

Smoking and Cancer Risk

He who saves a single life, it is as if he saved the world. Talmud

Cigarette smoking has many effects on your body, and one of the most feared is an increased risk of cancer. This chapter will review some basic information about cells to help you understand the effects smoking has on cells throughout your body and how cigarette smoking can lead to different forms of cancer.

Each cell in your body has an outer membrane that holds its contents in place. The liquid inside the cell, called the cytoplasm, contains different structures that perform the many functions of the cell. The nucleus of the cell contains the DNA (deoxyribonucleic acid) of your body organized into forty-six chromosomes and containing about 20,000 genes (Figure 8). These genes are DNA sequences that code for specific traits that are unique to you, such as hair and eye color, skin color, and your individual risk for certain diseases. The genetic risk for these diseases may also be found in your family history, such as having had a relative with diabetes, heart disease, cancer, or psychiatric disease (including addiction).

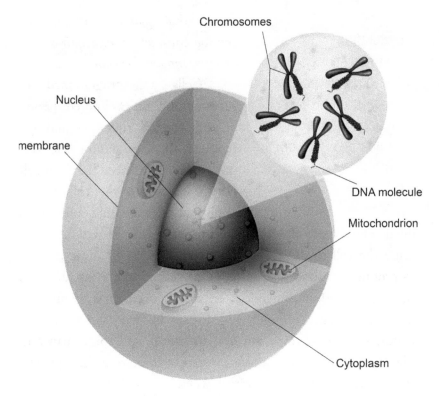

Figure 8: The cell, nucleus, and chromosomes.

When a cell divides, it makes a copy of its DNA and then splits the cell membrane to generate an exact copy of the original cell. Every day, millions of new cells are produced, and every day millions of cells die. But not all cells are the same. For example, millions of blood cells are produced on a daily basis at an incredibly fast rate. In contrast, nerve cells replicate at a very slow rate. All of this division is programmed by your DNA, which is the master blueprint for all cellular activity.

With all of this birth and death and replication of cells, errors and breaks in the DNA will naturally occur. A sophisticated system of DNA repair and surveillance is constantly working to identify DNA errors and fix them from the strands of DNA in each of your chromosomes. If a genetic error occurs and isn't repaired, a mutation has developed that could alter the cell's function. A mutation is an abnormal sequence of DNA that can be inherited

> "A mutation is an abnormal sequence of DNA that can be inherited from your parents, or can be spontaneous, or can be acquired from an environmental exposure."

from your parents, or can be spontaneous, *or can be acquired from an environmental exposure.*

Cells are programmed to survive only for a limited period of time before they die and get replaced. If a mutation overrode the genetic sequences that controls normal lifespan for that cell, the cell might not die and could continue to divide many times and form into a cancer. Other mutations might cause the cell to die faster than normal or might cause the cell to produce an abnormal protein that was critical to its function. In other situations, a random error may occur in a segment of DNA that doesn't seemingly code for any known process. In other words, some mutations can lead to cancer and some may not. The surveillance system that's constantly correcting these genetic mutations doesn't perform as well when we get older.

Cigarette Smoking and the Risk of Cancer

When you smoke cigarettes, tar is deposited in your mouth, throat, and lungs, and it coats the cells in those locations. Tar is the real culprit in cigarette-associated cancer risk, and it is the thick, molasses-like byproduct of tobacco smoke that contains about seventy known carcinogens. **A carcinogen is a chemical that can cause cancer.** Tar is like the cargo plane that distributes these carcinogens to multiple tissues in your body, and the concentration is highest on surfaces it lands on, including the mouth, throat, and lungs, when you inhale cigarette smoke. You'll swallow some of this tar as well, exposing your esophagus and stomach to it. Chemicals in tar also enter the bloodstream and get distributed around the body. Nicotine and tar are the two main components of cigarettes, and nicotine (described in Chapter Fourteen) is an intensely addictive substance which by itself is not considered to be cancer causing. At least twenty of the carcinogens in tar, listed in Table 1, have been directly and individually shown to cause lung tumors in at least one species of laboratory animal.

Carcinogen Class	Carcinogen Chemical Name
Polycyclic aromatic hydrocarbons	Benzo[*a*]pyrene
	Benzo[*b*]fluoranthene
	Benzo[*j*]fluoranthene
	Benzo[*k*]fluoranthene
	Dibenzo[*a,i*]pyrene
	Indeno[1,2,3-*cd*]pyrene
	Dibenz[*a,h*]anthracene
	5-Methylchrysene
Asz-arenes	Dibenz[*a,h*]acridine
	7H-Dibenzo[*c,g*]carbazole
N-Nitrosamines	*N*-Nitrosodiethylamine
	4-(Methylnitrosamino)-1-(3-pyridyl)-1-butanone (NNK)
Miscellaneous organic compounds	1,3-Butadiene
	Ethyl carbamate
Inorganic compounds	Nickel
	Chromium
	Cadmium
	Polonium-210
	Arsenic
	Hydrazine

Table 1: Carcinogens in Cigarette Smoke.

Adapted from International Agency for Research on Cancer (IARC) Working Group on the Evaluation of Carcinogenic Risks to Humans: 2004.

Imagine these dozens of carcinogens interacting with your mouth, throat, and lung cells every day. Changes and mutations are bound to occur. Let's focus on dibenzopyrene from this list as one example of how it affects DNA repair. This chemical is found in tar. Its byproducts can directly bind to the DNA molecule to form a DNA adduct: a segment of DNA bound to a cancer-causing chemical. This change in the DNA structure can directly cause a mutation in the area where the carcinogen from tar is attached. The DNA in this region can't be properly repaired back to its original sequence due to the adduct, resulting in a new mutation. This new mutation gets passed on to the next generation of cells. If this mutation occurs in a gene coding for normal cellular growth, the result could be abnormal growth and possibly cancer. If a mutation occurs in a gene that **suppresses** cancer growth, the result of removing this brake on cancer growth could also be cancer.

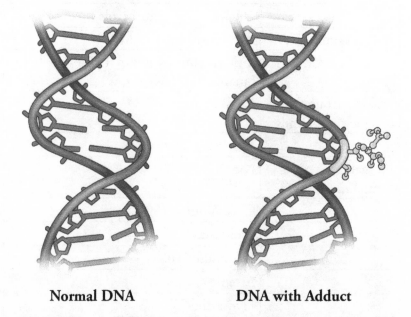

Normal DNA   **DNA with Adduct**

Figure 9: DNA adducts.

Just as there are many carcinogens, there are many different mechanisms in which the carcinogens in tar can cause cancer. Acetaldehyde is another carcinogen found in cigarette tar, and it can directly bind to the DNA molecule, also forming a DNA adduct. Alcohol is broken down into the carcinogen acetaldehyde, and this is one of the reasons alcohol use is associated with cancer.

If you imagine how many carcinogens are constantly binding randomly to your cells' DNA and having a cumulative effect over time, you'll understand how much **genetic chaos** this causes. All of these mutations certainly increase your risk of cancer, but they don't guarantee that any one person will get cancer. Perhaps mutations occur but are all largely successfully repaired. Or perhaps a mutation happens in a region of DNA that isn't important for cancer risk. It's very random, and just because your mother or father didn't get cancer from smoking is no protection for your future.

Recent data in lung cancer research has shown how common mutations are in smokers. This research also found that *entire regions of chromosomes* can be *completely deleted* in the early forms of many lung cancers associated with smoking. That's extraordinary evidence of the damaging effect of smoking on your DNA.

DNA is like a massive molecular zipper, constantly unwinding and then rewinding to open and close to replicate itself perfectly millions of times every day. When zippers work perfectly, it's a smooth operation. What happens when something gets caught in a zipper and it can't function properly? This huge number of mutations explain why cancers develop from these random and preventable errors caused by smoking-associated carcinogens.

Table 2 lists cancers that are linked to smoking and the relative risk of getting these cancers over an extended exposure to regular cigarette smoking compared to nonsmokers. Relative risk (RR) is the likelihood of an event occurring in an exposed group versus an unexposed group. If the RR is 1, the risk is the same between the two groups. If the RR is 2, the risk of getting that cancer in a smoker is twice as high (or 100 percent higher)

"Relative risk (RR) is the likelihood of an event occurring in an exposed group versus an unexposed group."

compared to a non-smoker. If the RR is 10, the risk of getting that cancer is ten times higher (or 1,000 percent higher).

Lung cancer has the highest risk, and this clear association between smoking and lung cancer was the basis of the *U.S. Surgeon General's Report* in 1964, commissioned by President Kennedy. This report clearly linked cigarette smoking with lung cancer. The first small health warnings began to appear on packs of cigarettes in 1965. In the fifty years since the Surgeon General's report, more data and hundreds of studies have linked cigarette smoke exposure to throat, esophageal, pancreatic, bladder, and other cancers.

Cancer Site	Average Relative Risk
Lung	15.0–30.0
Larynx	10.0*
Oral cavity	4.0–5.0
Oropharynx and hypopharynx	4.0–5.0*
Esophagus	1.5–5.0*
Pancreas	2.0–4.0
Urinary tract	3.0
Bladder	2.6–5.7
Nasal cavity, sinuses, nasopharynx	1.5–2.5
Stomach	1.5–2.0
Liver	1.5–2.5
Kidney	1.5–2.0
Uterine cervix	1.5–2.5
Myeloid leukemia	1.5–2.0

Table 2: Cigarette Smoking and Cancer Risk.

*Combined interaction with alcohol increases the risk; data from Vineis P et al, 2004.

The risk of some of these cancers, like esophageal cancer, is worsened by exposure to both cigarettes and alcohol. Bladder cancer is known to be associated with cigarette smoking because cancer causing chemicals are concentrated in the urine, where it sits in the bladder causing changes in bladder cells even though these cells aren't directly exposed to cigarette smoke.

Of the cancers in Table 2, lung cancer remains one of the deadliest, as you can understand from the story of Roger Sako in Chapter Two. Anthony Ficaro in Chapter Seven developed non-small cell lung cancer. Because of the huge global epidemic of cigarette use in the twentieth century, lung cancer is now estimated to be the most common cause of cancer death in the world. There are more patients dying with lung cancer each year in the U.S. (148,869 in 2018) than deaths from breast, colon, and prostate cancers *combined*.

> "Lung cancer is now estimated to be the most common cause of cancer death in the world."

Lung cancer is divided into two main categories:

- **Small-cell lung cancer** accounts for about 20 percent of all cases. As Roger's story describes, it is a cancer that quickly travels to brain and bone and is only rarely cured by surgery. While small cell lung cancer might initially respond to chemotherapy, with improvement in symptoms and quality of life, the majority of patients have a survival that can be measured in months, and they suffer from shortness of breath, cough, pain, weakness, and poor appetite.
- **Non-small cell lung cancer** has several subtypes and is more prone to grow locally before it begins to spread outside the lung.

Lung cancer, especially small cell lung cancer, is highly prone to spread around the body. This process is called **metastasis**—the ability of cancer cells to leave their primary tissue and invade or travel to other tissues.

For lung cancer overall, only 18 percent of people (on average) are alive five years after diagnosis. For this reason, it is crucial to prevent the development of lung cancer by preventing

teenage initiation of smoking, and by helping smokers quit
successfully as soon as possible.

There are some glimmers of hope in the relatively short
history of lung cancer—a disease that was actually rare before the
epidemic of smoking in the twentieth century as seen in Figure 10.
In the late 1800s, before cigarettes were factory manufactured and
easily available in large quantities, lung cancer was rare. Finding a
lung cancer during an autopsy back then was uncommon. Smoking
rates increased dramatically in the 1920s and only began to slowly
decline in the United States years after the first Surgeon General's
report on smoking was published in 1964.

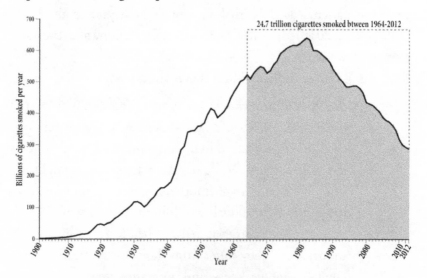

The Health Consequences of Smoking:
50 Years of Progress. A Report of the Surgeon General.

Figure 10: Total Cigarette Consumption, United States 1900-2012

U.S. Department of Health and Human Services, 2014, with permission

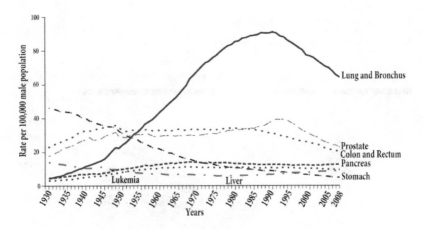

Figure 11: Mortality Rates From Selected Cancers Among Men in the United States, 1930-2008

U.S. Department of Health and Human Services, 2014, with permission

The epidemic of lung cancer death in women shown in **Figure 12** was also very clear late in the twentieth century, although women's peak rates were lower than in men due to lower rates of smoking among women.

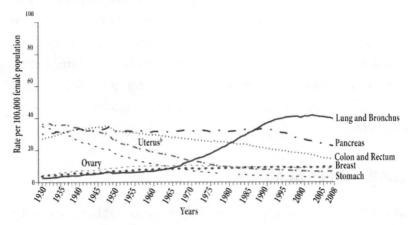

Figure 12: Mortality Rates In Selected Cancers Among Women in the United States, 1930-2008

U.S. Department of Health and Human Services, 2014, with permission

Figure 13 shows the distribution of lung cancer deaths by state in 2014. The darkest colors have the highest death rates. You can see that the highest lung cancer death rates were in the Southeast and other pockets around the United States.

Deaths from Lung Cancer by State

Rates of dying from lung cancer also vary from state to state.

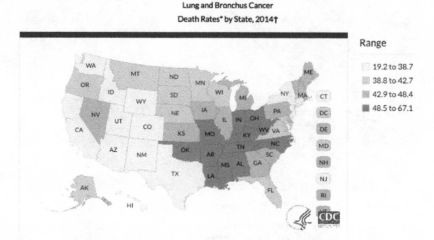

Figure 13. Deaths From Lung Cancer by State in the United States.

From the Centers for Disease Control and Prevention, 2018, with permission

Today, approximately 90 percent of all lung cancers are due to cigarette smoking, making it the most preventable cancer. That is a truly remarkable fact to understand—lung cancer was once rare and is now the leading cause of cancer death in the United States. Lung cancer, however, does not have to be your potential fate, and your risk of lung cancer can be significantly lowered by quitting cigarettes.

Lung Cancer Screening

In the past, doctors have not routinely screened for lung cancer the way they do for other cancers, like cervical cancer (with the **Pap smear**), breast cancer (with the **mammogram**), or prostate cancer (with the **PSA test**). The National Cancer Institute studied screening for lung cancer with chest x-rays and sputum tests in male smokers in the 1980s and found no benefit for reducing deaths from lung cancers detected with these tests. Without screening, most smokers who develop lung cancer see a physician only when the tumor is large enough to cause pain, weight loss, increased cough, blood in their sputum, or other symptoms. Early non-small lung cancers remain small and stay in place for years without causing symptoms until eventually they become large enough (often the size of a lemon or larger) to cause discomfort. Except for the airways, lung tissue itself is relatively insensitive, and slow-growing tumors may not cause symptoms for a long time.

Without screening, less than 20 percent of people who get lung cancer have it caught in an early stage—the rest have locally advanced or metastatic disease that has traveled beyond the small area a surgeon can remove in an attempt to cure the patient.

In 2011, the National Lung Screening Trial (NLST) was completed and reported that chest CT scan screenings for regular smokers that were fifty-five years of age or older **can detect lung cancer in its earliest stages and improve overall survival**. A CT scan is a quick and painless test found in all local hospitals, and it's better for detecting small changes in lung tissue than an x-ray. This new screening tool is now recommended by the American Cancer Society and is increasingly covered by insurance plans. For a screening tool (like mammography for breast cancer) to become widely used, it needs to be cost effective, and this has been demonstrated in the trial for CT scan screening for lung cancer. We cannot fully predict which smokers will get lung cancer, so prevention of smoking and early smoking cessation combined with early detection is thought to have the biggest impact on reducing the risk of death from lung cancer for the average cigarette smoker. **Talk to your doctor about lung cancer screening.**

How Quitting Reduces Cancer Risk

The good news is that quitting will dramatically reduce your lifetime risk of getting lung and other cancers. The sooner you quit, the more time you will give your body to heal and begin to reverse the damage and mutations that have formed. Many of the mutations found in the airways of most smokers are reversible. So the earlier

"So the earlier you quit, the more benefit you get. You will experience a reduced cancer risk with smoking cessation."

you quit, the more benefit you get. You will experience a reduced cancer risk with smoking cessation—do not think it's too late. Not only will you receive this benefit from quitting, you will also reduce your risk of lung and heart disease as you take control of your health.

To review, your cells are constantly dividing, and a sophisticated DNA repair system is in place in your body to correct any mutations that occur. Just as sun exposure can increase your risk of skin cancer, cigarette smoking is an environmental exposure that can cause mutations in your DNA and increase your risk of lung cancer and other cancers. There are multiple cancers associated with smoking, but the highest risk is lung cancer, which is the leading cause of cancer death in the United States. Recent research has demonstrated that lung cancer screening with CT scans is capable of catching lung cancer earlier and improving the chances for survival. Hundreds of clinical trials are evaluating many new therapies for lung cancer and other tobacco-related cancers. Once you stop smoking, your cancer risk diminishes with time. Because this risk reduction takes years to have its greatest benefit, it's important that you quit smoking as soon as possible.

What You Need to Know

- Approximately one-third of all cancers are caused by cigarette smoking. Smoking is the leading cause of preventable cancer.

- The tar in cigarettes has about 70 different chemical carcinogens that are distributed throughout your body when you smoke.

- Carcinogens you inhale cause changes in the DNA in your cells. These mutations can turn normal cells into cancer cells.

- Lung cancer is the most common tobacco-related cancer. It's the leading cause of death from cancer in the world, and in 2018, it still had only an 18 percent survival rate five years after diagnosis.

- Stopping smoking will reduce your risk of cancer—the sooner you stop, the greater the benefit.

CHAPTER FOURTEEN

Nicotine and Your Brain

Life is a sum of all your choices. So what are you doing today? **Albert Camus**

As you think about quitting and the options available to help you, it makes sense to step back and understand nicotine and why it's so addictive. You can walk into many pharmacies or chain stores and buy nicotine patches or gum and start using them right away without much thought or preparation. If you use patches or gum without any additional support, new studies suggest that you are less likely to be successful at quitting smoking than the people who received these medications in a clinical trial. This is likely due to a combination of a lack of support, incorrect use of the nicotine-replacement therapy, and the lack of an unclear plan; that's why things fall apart when you hit a challenge. Using medication without a good plan can be discouraging and might make you think you cannot quit. Nothing could be further from the truth, and this chapter will explain why. Each smoker in this book has a unique relationship with nicotine, and so do you.

If you plan to climb a mountain, your success involves preparation, understanding the terrain, gathering tools, and setting up a plan and supplies. The process of preparation can provide confidence—you see the issue before you—you've done some homework, set a course, and packed that final bag with the sense that you're ready. Success requires **knowledge**, **confidence**, and **motivation**. All three together creates the strongest combination for the best long-term results.

Each person in this book has climbed that summit successfully—don't defeat yourself by saying it can't be done. All successful scientists, inventors, and explorers know that failure is essential to success—they started with a vision of their destination and committed to it, even through failures and setbacks. The key is to *actively learn from setbacks* and then make modifications before continuing the journey. Quitting smoking is the most important thing you will ever do for your health.

> "Quitting smoking is the most important thing you will ever do for your health."

One of the biggest obstacles in your path is nicotine addiction; this chapter will discuss nicotine and why it is so addictive.

What Is Nicotine?

Nicotine is a highly water-soluble chemical that is rapidly absorbed and delivered directly to your brain within five heartbeats when you smoke. Your lungs have roughly the surface area of a tennis court. Smoking a cigarette delivers nicotine over that large surface, where it's rapidly absorbed into the bloodstream and delivered in seconds directly to your brain. Nicotine is a chemical that's similar in structure to a critically important chemical in your brain called **acetylcholine**—a key neurotransmitter that allows brain cells to communicate. Brain cells are highly interconnected, and they communicate by sending chemical messages to one other. Nicotine from outside your body begins to override this system, and your brain becomes dependent on it.

Nicotine binds to receptors on brain cells, causing a flood of chemical reactions and responses, including the release of **dopamine**—the pleasure chemical. This means that with every puff of a cigarette, your brain gets a message of pleasure and reward, leaving you wanting more. This helps to explain why some cigarettes really enhance the reward signals we get from pleasurable events like a great meal or sex. Nicotine can enhance your mood, concentration, and performance. In other situations, the feeling of reward you get is relief from the stress or anxiety of nicotine withdrawal if your nicotine level is low. Nicotine helps to relieve the symptoms of nicotine-withdrawal syndrome.

Your cigarette is the delivery vehicle of nicotine, and nicotine stimulates your reward center—it's that simple.

Do you remember the first cigarette you ever smoked? It likely caused you to be suddenly dizzy, perhaps mildly nauseated. Saliva might have pooled in your mouth. Whatever your reaction to the first time you smoked, it was *fast* and intense, and then it took a while to feel normal again. Years later, when you are a regular smoker, your reaction to a cigarette is never as intense. The reason is that your brain structure changes with regular smoking by increasing the number of receptors for nicotine. In **Figure 14**, you can see the low staining of nicotinic receptors in the brain of a non-smoker (picture A). In picture B you can see that the concentration of nicotinic receptors is much higher. **This is direct evidence that nicotinic receptors and your brain structure are changed by smoking cigarettes.** The same mechanism is likely true if you vape nicotine. Once this has happened, you may need months for your brain chemistry to return to a more normal state.

Temporal Cortex

A. Nonsmoker

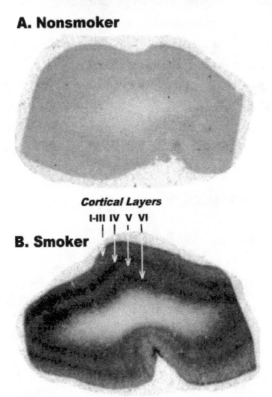

Cortical Layers
I-III IV V VI

B. Smoker

Figure 14: Increased nicotinic receptors in the brain of smokers

From Perry et al, 1999, with permission.

Nicotine is similar to the addiction potential of cocaine and heroin. All three drugs share the same addictive properties by stimulating the release of dopamine from your brain's pleasure center. **Figure 15** shows that there's a concentrated part of the brain that's activated with exposure to nicotine. It causes the release of dopamine in the reward center. By smoking cigarettes, you've tapped in to one of the most important and primitive centers in your brain and hit the override switch. Many smokers started experimenting with cigarettes as teenagers, misunderstanding or ignoring how addictive it is. The faster nicotine is absorbed, the more addictive it is, and delivering nicotine to the lungs by smoking or vaping is extraordinarily fast and effective at getting it into your brain. Cocaine smoked as crack is more addictive than cocaine snorted into your nose because it's so rapidly and efficiently absorbed in the lungs, which have a larger surface area than your sinuses and cause faster absorption.

In comparison, nicotine delivered by a skin patch, gum, or lozenge is absorbed at a slower rate, generating a nicotine level lower than that of smoking. This explains why nicotine patches, gum, and lozenges have a very low-to-no addiction potential.

Your Brain on Nicotine

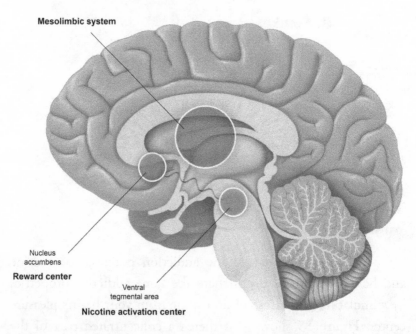

Figure 15: The reward center releasing dopamine in the brain when it's activated by nicotine.

Nicotine has a half-life of two hours, meaning that half of it is gone from your bloodstream in two hours (**Figure 16**). This is very fast! People who metabolize nicotine faster than others need higher doses to stay in the pleasure and arousal zone and will subsequently smoke more cigarettes. By the time you wake up in the morning, your nicotine level has dropped very low or even to zero. Many people smoke a couple of cigarettes quickly to get their blood levels back up to feel better or treat intense morning cravings. Does this happen to you? This spike in nicotine happens multiple times during the day with regular smoking, with more pleasure or satisfaction or arousal after a cigarette and then a drop in nicotine levels leading to more discomfort and an urge when the nicotine level gets too low.

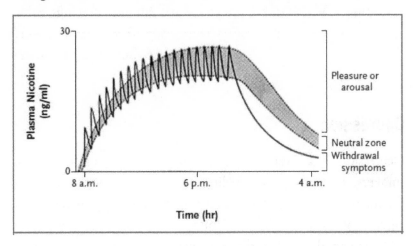

Figure 16: Nicotine levels in a smoker consuming one pack of 20 cigarettes.

Nicotine levels in a smoker consuming one pack of 20 cigarettes; From Benowitz, 2010, with permission.

Nicotine Withdrawal

Nicotine *withdrawal* symptoms can include irritability, depressed mood, restlessness and/or anxiety. Think about this for a minute— once a smoker has become addicted to nicotine, he or she frequently smokes to avoid these negative symptoms, which can be very unpleasant and intense. These withdrawal symptoms and urges are especially powerful because your brain has developed a chemical dependency over time, and it will take some time (months) to revert the brain back to its original balance. In other words, sudden withdrawal of nicotine from a nicotine-addicted brain can feel like an acute psychiatric illness. Nicotine in the form of cigarettes or e-cigarettes is readily available in almost every

"Think about this for a minute—once a smoker has become addicted to nicotine, he or she frequently smokes to avoid these negative symptoms, which can be very unpleasant and intense."

corner store and supermarket and gas station. This easy availability makes it that much harder for you to escape nicotine. Be aware that this substance is extraordinarily potent and be very mindful of its effect on you. It's not your fault that you have intense cravings when you're away from cigarettes—it's the response your brain has when it doesn't get nicotine.

Depression

Depression is an especially important issue to understand in smokers. Depression is a feeling of sadness or hopelessness, or the inability to enjoy things that others enjoy. Approximately 10 percent of all adults in the United States have been diagnosed with major depressive disorder over a twelve-month period. These rates are higher in young adults and higher in women than in men. Depression is caused by an imbalance in your brain's neurotransmitters, especially dopamine and serotonin, and both of these chemicals are changed by cigarette smoking. Research has revealed that tar in cigarettes has a chemical that's actually an antidepressant. This effect is separate from the way nicotine changes your neurotransmitter balance. In other words, both tar and nicotine can have antidepressant effects. Smokers with depression understandably have a harder time quitting. *If you have depression you can quit successfully.* Studies have shown that smokers with depression have improvement in their depression after quitting.

If you started smoking as a teenager, you can see the impact that nicotine can have on your behavior. What if you were prone to depression and began to experiment with cigarettes or e-cigarettes? What if you found that they seemed to help your depression? You become addicted to them and realize that you have to smoke more cigarettes over time to get the same effect. This is called **tolerance: when you need higher doses of a drug to feel the same effect** because your brain structure has changed. Tolerance is also seen in other addictions, like opioid or alcohol abuse.

If you stop smoking cold turkey, you feel terrible. Will you have depression, or just experience nicotine withdrawal? The answer is that you might have both. This is a situation where it's especially important to talk to a health-care provider because symptoms of depression can be treated. Depression might influence the choice of smoking-cessation medications that will work best for you. Your symptoms of depression can be measured over time to see if you have an underlying depression or not, and depression is very treatable.

What You Need to Know

- Nicotine is a highly potent, mind-altering chemical found in tobacco.
- Nicotine is powerful because it mimics acetylcholine—one of the most common chemicals in your brain. Exposure to nicotine changes your brain chemistry.
- After repeated exposure, the brain gets used to regular nicotine doses and causes intense symptoms of withdrawal if nicotine levels drop too low.
- Nicotine is metabolized quickly in the body. People who metabolize it faster than others need higher doses to stay in the pleasure and arousal zone and will subsequently smoke more cigarettes.

- The more you understand nicotine, the greater the likelihood that you'll be able to overcome nicotine addiction.

CHAPTER FIFTEEN

Medications and How They're Used in Smoking Cessation

I never lose. I either win or learn. **Nelson Mandela**

Many people successfully stop smoking using medications, either over the counter or with a prescription or both. Even so, there are plenty of smokers who elect to quit cold turkey, meaning without any medication or counseling support. It's important to explore which methods you're drawn to use, because any decision will be more effective if it's a conscious decision you've made for yourself. To make an informed choice, it's important to know how medications are used.

Another key to success is the willingness to be adaptable and flexible. In other words, make your choices in the spirit of **exploration**. Make a plan, put it in motion and then assess how it's going. If what you set in place isn't working as you would like, be willing to make changes to your plan. For example, if you decide to use the nicotine patch and find that certain situations and intense urges make it difficult to not pick up a cigarette, you could consider adding a short-acting nicotine replacement to your nicotine patch program for breakthrough urges. You should evaluate which situations are especially challenging, and why. Developing a plan was covered in Chapters Nine and Ten. Try to remain committed to your plan and be able to change it rather than abandon it.

"Only about one-third of smokers making a quit attempt use the very important and effective medications options available."

One of the first questions you might have about a quit plan is whether you want to use any medication at all. If it's important to you to try to quit cold turkey, this can be your first plan. Be prepared to reassess using medications if it turns out that going cold turkey does not work for you. The cold turkey method is not very effective, so if it fails, do not start to believe that you can't quit. High-quality research has shown that smoking-cessation medications are effective. We recommend them to increase the likelihood of your success. Despite the benefits seen with either counseling or medication, only about one-third of smokers making a quit attempt use either of these important and effective options. This is unfortunate because it means people are less likely to get the huge benefit that comes with stopping smoking.

People often approach smoking-cessation medications with different ideas and preferences. Consider these issues carefully in advance of your quit date to feel fully committed to a plan. All of the medications approved for use by the regulatory agencies, such as the Food & Drug Administration (FDA) have been determined to be safe and effective. Each medication has a different delivery method (eg. transdermal patch vs lozenge). These medications decrease nicotine-withdrawal symptoms, so you are free to make behavioral changes that will keep you off cigarettes.

Now that you understand how nicotine is delivered in cigarettes and how it affects your brain (Chapter Fourteen), it might make more sense to you why providing **Nicotine Replacement Therapy (NRT)**, which is gradually lowered over months, is a good way to help smokers quit. The replacement therapies provide lower levels of nicotine without the harmful tar. They have helped millions of people around the world quit and stay quit.

Choosing a cessation medication is a personal decision about what is the right choice for you. Take some time reading this chapter and be aware of the benefits and risks before starting. Talk to your health-care provider or a pharmacist if you still have questions. Many medications are available over the counter without a doctor's prescription, and the cost is about the same as paying for a pack of cigarettes a day. Many insurance plans will cover even over the counter medications if you have a prescription. Cessation medications are designed to be used for a few months or possibly longer as necessary. Even if the initial cost is similar to or a bit higher than smoking, once you stop successfully, the financial savings will start to add up. The health benefits start right away.

There is an important difference between "clean" and "dirty" nicotine, as people sometimes refer to them.

- **Clean nicotine** is synthesized by licensed and regulated pharmaceutical manufacturers and compounded into a gum or a patch without any of the carcinogenic tar found in cigarettes.

- **Dirty nicotine** is in cigarettes and cigars and in any tobacco product. E-cigs contain dirty nicotine because it is turned into vapor along with other chemicals and metals in the heating coil. Breathing in these metals along with high levels of nicotine is potentially harmful.

If having any nicotine in your system after your quit date concerns you, perhaps this difference will help you move toward the clean nicotine found in NRT, like nicotine gum, the patch, lozenges, inhalers, and nasal spray. If you want to completely leave all nicotine behind, there are other options available for you, like oral medications.

No medication will completely reduce all urges to smoke. You need to have strategies for handling urges after your quit date.

Ask your doctor or nurse to see what they may be able to advise; pharmacists can be a great resource as well. Ideally, if you can identify a **smoking cessation specialist** or a **Certified Tobacco Treatment Specialist (CTTS)**, you will have found someone who is fully informed about all current treatment options.

It's worth stressing the importance of flexibility. You might start a quit plan and then find that it's not working as you had hoped. This is part of learning to quit—it is not failure. You can potentially add two or more medications together or make other adjustments to your plan to make it more effective. This is a time when having a good relationship with a health-care provider can be helpful as you navigate your way to success. If you feel you don't have a good relationship with a nurse or doctor or pharmacist, take the time *now* to build one and don't give up until you're satisfied.

Nicotine Replacement Therapies

Nicotine replacement therapies are effective and safe ways to help you quit smoking. They can lower urges to smoke that you experience after your quit date. These therapies are listed in Table 4 and they have two issues in common:

1. They are absorbed into the bloodstream at a slower rate than a cigarette.

2. Their peak nicotine level is typically lower than the level you get from smoking a cigarette.

Why is this important? Understanding these two issues will help you anticipate that using them will *reduce* the number and intensity of urges you would experience with smoking, but they will not *eliminate* the urges. NRTs typically cannot give you the same nicotine exposure you had as a smoker, and, therefore, you will still have cravings. With time, measured in weeks, the number and intensity of these cravings will decrease.

Nicotine Replacement Therapies (NRTs)

Replacement Therapy	Route of Administration	Availability	Side Effects
Nicotine patch	Skin—transdermal delivery	OTC and prescription	Skin reaction at site of use, insomnia, or unusual dreams
Nicotine gum	Oral—chewed and parked between cheek and gums	OTC and prescription	Jaw soreness, loose fillings, heartburn, nausea, hiccups
Nicotine lozenge	Oral	OTC and prescription	Heartburn, nausea, hiccups
Nicotine inhaler	Oral—mouth exposure with quick puffs	Prescription only	Sore throat
Nicotine nasal spray	Nasal spray	Prescription only	Headache, runny nose and eyes

Table 4: Nicotine Replacement Therapies (NRTs)

*OTC , over the counter

As you think about these options, what appeals to you? Which seem the most familiar? Have you or a friend used any of them in the past? What was it like? Because the effectiveness seen with these NRTs is about the same, the one that seems the best to *you* is a great place for you to start because you're most likely to use it regularly and correctly. If you've used an NRT in the past successfully and for an extended period of time, it might be the best method to use again. It's already familiar to you and has been proven successful for you, and you can use it with confidence.

If the NRT or other medication worked well, focus on why you relapsed and develop a plan for this. For example, a woman I know who recently received advice on quitting chose a medication and was successful for a few months. It was easier than she thought it would be, but she found the idea of driving without smoking extremely difficult and eventually relapsed. In this case, it's clear that the medication had its desired effect, but that she would benefit from specific ideas to help her drive without smoking.

Success rates at twelve months are approximately 20 percent to 30 percent with NRT. This is dramatically higher than going cold turkey (2 percent to 4 percent success at twelve months). Don't let these statistics scare you. You're primed for success with all of the information and advice in this book. That puts you ahead of the pack. In clinical trials the NRT was more effective than placebo, proving that the method is effective. The key to successful quitting is the knowledge that it's difficult and requires your focus and commitment *over the long term*—if it were easy, success rates would be much higher.

> "Different people need different strategies."

These quit rates tell us that success is attainable, but it's not due to the medication alone. Different people need different strategies. Consider a motivated pregnant woman smoking half a pack per day versus the struggle faced by a two-pack-per-day middle-aged man with depression and alcoholism. There's no one-size-fits-all strategy, and drop-out rates (which count as failure) in clinical studies of cessation medications are often high.

The Mayo Clinic website has reliable information on NRTs and other therapies; it's a good place to go if you're looking for additional resources (https://www.mayoclinic.org; search "quit-smoking products"). If medical care is available to you, you should talk with your doctor or nurse about the pros and cons of NRTs and review all package inserts, which cover use and precautions for each of these medications. There are specific precautions about the use of NRT in people that have had a recent heart attack or have abnormal heart rhythms or angina (heart pain). The package inserts are available online and have all of the prescribing information you need (or you can ask your doctor's staff to print them for you).

In our experience, *an important issue with NRTs is that they're often used incorrectly.* You should always buy a supply of NRT before your quit date, and, ideally, you should take them to your doctor or pharmacist to carefully go over their proper use.

Nicotine Patches

Nicotine patches should be put on in the morning as soon as you get up. If you have a regular morning routine that includes cigarettes, change this routine by putting on the patch first. You can wear one in the shower or bath as long as it's has been well placed (pressed firmly for thirty seconds on skin that is not hairy, is well dried, and that is not covered in lotion). There are different doses of nicotine patches, and the dose may vary based on your level of nicotine addiction and the amount you smoke. Be sure to read the instructions carefully to use them properly. If you have symptoms of insomnia or bad dreams, the patch should be taken off at night. A new patch should be applied to a different location on your body every twenty-four hours. Never cut a patch in half— cutting makes them ineffective because the nicotine in the gel of the patch evaporates.

Patches are designed to maintain a constant level of nicotine during the day and are then reduced in dose over months. The intent is that they will prevent strong urges. They must be used every single day during this time. If you would typically smoke a few cigarettes in the morning as you get up, this pattern of smoking suggests that a short-acting NRT, like a lozenge or gum or inhaler, *with or without the patch,* might get you through the time it takes for the nicotine level from the patch in your bloodstream to rise.

Sometimes, people who do well on the patch become overconfident after several weeks of not smoking. They stop using the patch too soon, assuming that it is no longer needed. In fact, they have not given their brains enough time to gradually adjust to this state of low nicotine exposure, and, without the patch, they have intense urges and are at risk to go back to smoking. It may take several months to be ready to stop using an NRT, and the clinical trials that have shown these medications are effective used NRT over months.

Short-acting NRTs: Over the Counter Gum and Lozenges

Gum or **lozenges** should be used regularly during the day *every one to two hours if they're the only cessation medications you're using.* Short-acting nicotine replacement is designed to *prevent* as well as to treat urges. The intent of these short-acting NRTs is to achieve a steady concentration of nicotine during the day, just as you did when you were smoking (see Figure 16 in Chapter Fourteen). **This makes regular dosing important, even when you are not experiencing an urge to smoke.**

Do not chew **nicotine gum** like ordinary chewing gum. The nicotine needs to be absorbed through the lining of your mouth, and from there into your blood stream where it can travel to the brain and prevent or provide relief from cravings. If the gum is chewed constantly, the nicotine will be released too quickly into the saliva and swallowed, where it will be neutralized by stomach acids and you will get no benefit from the nicotine. Nicotine in your stomach can lead to nausea and hiccups.

The correct way to use the gum is to chew it until you feel a tingling sensation or taste the flavor of the gum. This is a sign that the nicotine is being released and that *it is time to park the gum between your cheek and gums until that sensation subsides.* Over the next 30 minutes, alternate between chewing and parking the gum.

Prescription NRT: Nasal Spray and Oral Inhaler

These forms of NRT are available only by prescription. The **nasal spray** is used one-to-two times per hour and isn't recommended if you have sinus problems. The nasal spray is just sprayed into the nostril without sniffing it into your sinuses. It can cause symptoms like watery eyes or throat irritation. The **oral inhaler** can be especially helpful if you have a very intense oral fixation with cigarettes and want something to put in your mouth. You take short, sharp puffs of the nicotine vapor into your mouth, where the nicotine is absorbed in your cheeks or the back of your throat. The oral inhaler is not used like inhalers that are breathed deeply into the lungs. Like other short-acting NRT, it needs to be used regularly during the day, and the recommended dose is six to sixteen cartridges per day for six to twelve weeks. It can cause mouth or throat irritation.

Give It Time

Generally, people do not use NRTs long enough. A minimum of three months of use is recommended, and it's often useful to continue use for longer periods of time if needed. This is another time where it will be important to assess how ready you might be to step down your dosage or to stop using a medication. If you do decrease your dose and find that your cravings are too hard to manage, it is appropriate to increase your dose. Think of NRT as a medicine you are using to manage your cravings and dose accordingly. There is no shame in increasing a medication that is keeping you from smoking tobacco. If you experience new side effects, talk to your health-care provider right away. Keep in mind the three "rights" that will boost your chances of success: **right dose** (correct dose of patch or short-acting NRT), **right daily timing** (when and how often you take it) and **right length of time** (months, not weeks).

Plasma Nicotine Concentrations for Nicotine-Containing Products

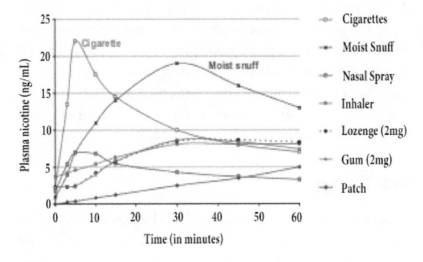

Figure 17: Nicotine levels over time using NRT

From RxForChange, 2006, with permission

In **Figure 17**, you can see that the initial peak nicotine level is higher with a cigarette and lower with all NRT. Of all of these, the patch is the slowest to increase nicotine in your bloodstream, but after an hour, it's comparable. Moist snuff is similar to the nasal spray in the first five minutes. Moist snuff is smokeless tobacco (also known as dip) that is not NRT, or a product called Snus, which is oral tobacco in pouches that is more frequently used as NRT in Europe.

Pregnancy

If you are pregnant, you may be highly motivated to quit. Smoking cessation during pregnancy is an important issue, and smoking is associated with low infant birth weight and increased risk of complications for both the mother and the baby. Pregnancy is a time when the motivation to become tobacco-free may be high, and motivation is a key factor in a successful plan. All efforts should be made to become tobacco-free, and studies show that counseling helps pregnant women quit. The evidence is strongest for using counseling without medication as a first option, and considering NRT, especially the patch, as a second option.

The safety of oral medications like varenicline or bupropion (discussed below) in pregnant women has not been fully established. It's critical that a quit plan and possible medication use be discussed with the health-care provider overseeing your pregnancy, and that you also talk to your doctor about the safety of using smoking-cessation medications during breast-feeding.

Oral Therapies

Two pill therapies (Table 5) are available by prescription and are approved by the U.S. FDA and other regulatory bodies around the world: **Zyban**® (Wellbutrin, bupropion SR) and **Chantix**® (varenicline). Both oral medications are designed to be taken for months. Zyban was first approved by the FDA in 1997 and is an antidepressant medication. It was noticed in clinical trials of depression that some patients taking the drug spontaneously quit smoking. It was then studied as a smoking-cessation drug. Zyban is the sustained release (SR) form of a medication called bupropion, which increases dopamine in your brain and is a dopamine and norepinephrine reuptake inhibitor. Zyban is now generic and helps to increase the level of dopamine in the brain. As you learned in Chapter Fourteen, dopamine is the pleasure chemical and one of the neurotransmitters released by cigarette smoking that makes nicotine so addictive.

Since the pill therapies for cessation take a while to have an effect, you will be directed to take the pills regularly *before your* quit date. The main effect of Zyban in people who have responded to it is a lower intensity and number of urges and less fixation on the next cigarette. Zyban is effective for smoking cessation in smokers with or without depression and is a logical choice in smokers with depression since it's an antidepressant. The quit rates for Zyban are higher than placebo or NRT when used as a single therapy, and *the combination of* Zyban *plus a nicotine patch is more successful than either one alone.*

Therapies - Pills

Oral Therapy	Effect	Dosing	Side Effects
Zyban (Wellbutrin, Bupropion SR)	Increased dopamine/ norepinephrine in the synapseth quick puffs	150 mg/day for 7 days, then 150 mg twice per day before and after quit date	Dry mouth, headache, insomnia, rare seizures, hypertension; neuropsychiatric reactions including suicidal thoughts; interactions with other drugs
Chantix (varenicline)	Dopamine release and nicotine blockade	0.5 mg/day for 3 days, then 0.5 mg twice daily for 4 days, followed by 1 mg twice/day	Nausea, vomiting, insomnia; neuropsychiatric side effects that might include agitation, depression, anxiety, or suicidal thoughts

Table 5: The Pills

Source: package inserts

The **Chantix®** (varenicline) pill was approved for smoking cessation in 2006. Chantix has the highest cessation rate, at six months. It binds a specific nicotinic receptor in the brain and causes dopamine release. It also prevents the binding of nicotine to that receptor. In this manner, it blunts the effect of nicotine from cigarettes and at the same time releases the main pleasure chemical (dopamine) that would be released by nicotine.

In theory, both the withdrawal effects from cessation are reduced, and the pleasure gained from smoking is reduced. Patients with significant psychiatric symptoms may be advised to not take Chantix, although studies are ongoing. Due to its potential psychological side effects, it is very important to review the information with your health-care provider. If you have any significant personality or mood changes, stop Chantix and contact your doctor or health care provider immediately.

Combination Therapy

An important trend in smoking-cessation medication strategies over the past ten years has been the use of **combination therapies**. Research shows specific medications, used in combination, can be more effective than therapies used alone. Because there are at least seven types of medication (five types of NRTs and two oral medications), the actual number of options that could be effective is large. This is good news. It might take several attempts before you find the option that has the biggest benefit for you. Combination therapies can also provide more flexibility in your plan, particularly if you start with one therapy, feel it's not fully effective, and want to add a second therapy. The range of options available today is much better than in the past.

"it might take several attempts before you find the option that has the biggest benefit for you."

One example to consider is the combination of nicotine patch and a short-acting NRT like nicotine gum. It can take close to sixty minutes before the nicotine absorbed from a patch reaches peak level. In comparison, it takes about thirty minutes for the gum to reach its peak. If you have strong nicotine withdrawal symptoms in the morning, combining the patch with gum could be a good solution. To do this effectively, you would wake up in the morning and immediately use a piece of gum and then place the nicotine patch as part of your normal morning routine. Research testing the patch versus gum versus the combination of patch and gum showed that the combination had a better cessation rate than either therapy alone.

Breakthrough urges could suggest that you are under-dosed by using only one patch (because people metabolize nicotine differently). The problem is under-dosing of nicotine, and the solution for some patients is to use more than one patch. Ernie Ring in Chapter Two chose to use more than one patch and found this to be successful. It is becoming more common for providers to consider

"Talk to your doctor or pharmacist about using increased doses of NRT or combining medications."

multiple patches or a combination of pills with NRT to help patients stop smoking. For example, a recent study concluded that the combination of Zyban and Chantix was more effective than either medication alone. All medications have side effects, and the combination of medications can have more side effects, but also the potential for more benefit. Talk to your doctor or pharmacist about using increased doses of NRT or combining medications.

Only the combination of Zyban and the nicotine patch has been formally approved by the FDA, but many other studies of combinations are ongoing and are not in the latest published smoking cessation guidelines. The most important point is that there is new data and great hope that you *can* quit with the right combination of behavioral change, motivation, and medication. Discuss these options with your health-care provider to determine if a combination of medications is a good choice for you.

Counseling

Many people who have addictions feel isolated and struggle talking about the problems they've experienced as they've tried to quit. This isolation could translate into a fear of joining smoking-cessation groups or being judged by others. Opening up, being more vocal, and listening to the struggles others face can provide you enormous energy and inspiration, which can be applied to your quit attempt. Opening up to other people, as the interviews in *Learning to Quit* have shown, is an important step in removing barriers to taking

> "If you have made a quit attempt and failed, it makes sense to explore counseling as a means of finding a different medication and staying on track."

action. There is a great benefit to receiving support and learning from others.

Both individual and group counseling are more effective than no counseling at all. If you have made a quit attempt and failed, it makes sense to explore counseling as a means of finding a different medication and staying on track. If you have been hospitalized, many hospitals offer in-hospital counseling, which is effective. Telephone counseling can improve quit rates, and free phone services are available nationally (like the CDC's phone service **1-800-QUITNOW**). If talking to your doctor about smoking increases your energy to quit, schedule a separate follow-up appointment to focus on this one specific issue. Too often, smokers are seen by a physician in a fifteen-minute visit and smoking is the last issue that's discussed. Tackling a significant challenge with a counselor or as part of a group can increase your energy level and significantly improve your chance of success. The people in this book were helped by reaching out and asking for support, and this option is worth serious consideration.

Vaping and Electronic Cigarettes

Electronic cigarettes (e-cigs) have become much more visible over the last ten years, and increasingly, tobacco companies are taking over this new market. We don't know if they're safe, and some research has shown that the super-heated metal coil in an e-cig releases metal vapors and other compounds that are directly toxic to airway cells in the lungs. The general assumption by the public is that e-cigs must be safer than cigarettes because they don't deliver the harmful tar that's described in Chapters Eleven and Thirteen. The recent epidemic of severe and fatal lung disease has made it clear that the safety of vaping is questionable.

A major concern in the public health community is

that vaping will be seen as an alternative to cigarette smoking in restaurants and bars and public places, reversing the incredibly hard work and progress over forty years that has gradually reduced cigarette use and tobacco-related disease in the United States and other countries. As you learned in Chapter Fourteen, *inhaled* nicotine is the most addictive form of nicotine. Vaping sustains nicotine addiction, and many people using e-cigs may not know that they're being exposed to nicotine. In 2005, approximately 2 percent of high school seniors admitted to using e-cigs, and by 2016 this number had climbed dramatically to 15 percent of high school seniors. In 2019, more than 25 percent of high school seniors reported vaping nicotine in the past thirty days.

"Inhaled nicotine is the **most addictive** form of nicotine."

There is now substantial evidence that eCig use increases the risk of using regular cigarettes among adolescents and young adults—a truly alarming trend. Among adolescents, eCig use is exploding globally, is unregulated, and is described as a public health disaster.

Here's an example the how the danger associated with vaping emerged. In 2018 in the journal *Pediatrics*. An 18-year-old woman tried vaping for the first time and shortly afterward had respiratory failure, requiring her to be placed on a breathing machine in the ICU of a local hospital. She had chest tubes surgically placed to remove fluid buildup around her lungs. The case report was one of several in the medical literature, but the first report concerning a teenager and it began to raise awareness.

Vaping was clearly unsafe for this young woman, and her story highlights how the safety of vaping has not been properly studied. Daily e-cigarette use has been independently associated with an increased risk of heart attack. Also of concern is the finding that the daily use of both e-cigarettes and cigarettes **together**, which is not uncommon, increases the risk of heart attack even further.

Limited research has been conducted with e-cigs as a smoking-cessation therapy. Several studies have suggested that vaping may have efficacy similar to that of nicotine patches. The only benefit to vaping found was that compliance might be better than the patch.

A recent trial was published in the *New England Journal of Medicine* in 2019 and compared NRT with e-cigarette use in a British study of close to nine hundred people. It's important to understand this trial because it made the most news and is frequently cited by the vaping industry. This was a randomized trial (which is good) but an unblinded trial (which is bad, because knowing which group you're in can artificially favor the e-cigarette group). The study showed that the one-year quit rate for NRT was 9.9 percent compared to the quit rate of 18 percent in the e-cigarette group.

While this might suggest that e-cigarettes have a place in smoking cessation, the study had a few major flaws:

A. It was not blinded, and this could cause people in the NRT group to lose motivation since they weren't getting the study "drug". The e-cig group might feel more motivated to quit.

B. Eighty percent of people in the e-cig group were still vaping at one year, compared to 9 percent in the NRT group, which stops NRT as directed after three to six months. This is very important because it suggests that e-cig users remain addicted to nicotine compared to NRT users who stopped smoking and also stopped NRT use.

C. The rate of quitting at one year for the e-cig group in this study is less than the published rate of quitting at one year for Zyban or Chantix, or the combination of Zyban and nicotine patch. The safety of these medications is understood, and the safety of vaping is not understood.

D. The whole objective of smoking cessation is to stop smoking and end nicotine addiction. Clearly, in this study, e-cigs did not accomplish this goal.

One of the biggest concerns we have with vaping is its addiction potential. The approach to smoking cessation is to take away the addicting cigarette and replace it with non-addictive alternatives over the course of several months. Using a patch or a pill for several months and then stopping is a better alternative to find a healthy new direction than vaping for an extended amount of time and not facing the primary nicotine addiction. There's a false narrative that since vaping may be safer than cigarettes, it must be safe. It would be much more accurate to say that vaping is likely less safe than nicotine replacement therapy, and that vaping has resulted in the addiction of a whole new generation that will suffer the financial, psychological, and harmful health consequences of chronic nicotine dependence.

In July and August of 2019, severe lung disease began to be reported from twenty-five states involving people that were vaping. This highlights what happens when companies producing a potentially dangerous substance aren't regulated and required to perform careful safety reporting. Many of these cases were linked to the use of THC (the active ingredient in marijuana) and might have been linked to additives that can cause severe lung inflammation when inhaled. Some of the cases were from e-cigarettes that used nicotine without THC.

Figure 18 shows you what a normal CT scan of the chest looks like. A CT scan means that the person is on his or her back while being moved forward onto a circular x-ray machine while image slices of the chest are then taken. CT scans have much finer detail than a regular chest x-ray. You can see that the heart in the middle, filled with blood, is dense and white, as the x-ray beams are reduced when they try to pass through the tissue. On the other hand, lung tissue, which is filled with air, is gray since x-ray beams pass right through it. You can see blood vessels in the lungs that show up as white lines because they're filled with blood and block the x-ray beams.

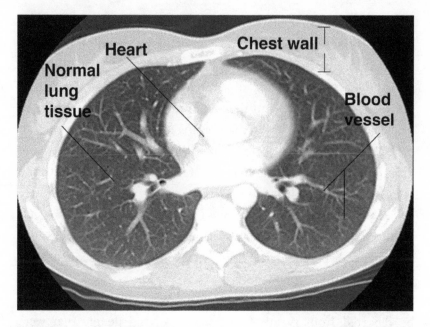

Figure 18: Normal CT scan of the chest

Case courtesy of A. Prof Frank Gaillard, Radiopaedia.org, rID: 8095

Now take a look at Figure 19—the chest CT image of a patient with vaping-associated lung disease. You can see that the normal lung tissue is now whiter and denser throughout both lungs. This represents serious lung tissue inflammation from the e-cigarette this person was using.

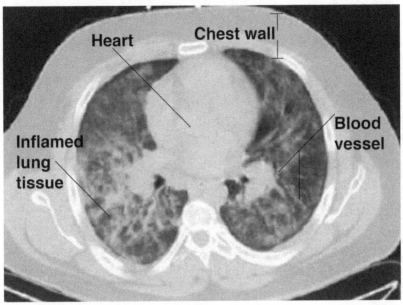

Figure 19: CT scan with severe lung inflammation from vaping

Image from CDC MMWR report, 2019

As of December 3, 2019, 2,291 cases of people with hospitalized e-cigarette or vaping acute lung injury (now called EVALI) have been reported from fifty states, Washington DC and two US territories. There have been forty-eight total deaths,with more deaths under investigation. The age range of people with lung injury is seventeen to seventy-five years old, and more than 50 percent of these people are less than twenty-five years of age. Lung transplants have been required in some people. The long term harm to lung health is only beginning to be studied.

To date, major medical societies do not recommend e-cigs for smoking cessation and instead have called for them to be regulated as cigarettes are and carefully studied. In light of the newly recognized epidemic of vaping-associated severe lung disease and deaths, e-cigarettes should not be used instead of regular cessation medications until both the short and long-term dangers associated with vaping are understood.

Alternative Interventions Such as Acupuncture and Hypnosis

Have you considered alternative options like acupuncture or hypnosis? Over the years, many people have tried or expressed an interest in these approaches. Because neither of these interventions has been formally tested, it's difficult to know how effective they are in comparison to other well-studied therapies. The delivery of these treatments is also highly variable and choosing a high-quality practitioner can be challenging. It's difficult to know if your practitioner is qualified and experienced. Hypnotherapy has been around for decades, and acupuncture has been in practice for centuries. We have heard from some of our participants that they have been helpful in stopping smoking.

We do not actively discourage someone from choosing either of these approaches. If you have committed to becoming smoke-free and become dedicated to these interventions, that's great news and deserving of support. We would recommend them in combination with a proven intervention like smoking-cessation medications and counseling. There are multiple websites that describe these services, and it is best to get a good recommendation before choosing a practitioner. **Everybody's journey is different, and the key is to learn from every action you take.**

Whatever path you choose, the key is to never stop trying, and to learn the most you can from each quit plan. If you dedicate yourself to learning to quit, you are much more likely to achieve the most important step you will ever take toward better health.

What You Need to Know

- There are two general classes of medications available to help you stop smoking: Nicotine Replacement Therapy and oral medications.

- Because these medications can be used either alone or in combination, there are multiple potential medication options available to you.

- You can significantly increase your chances of success if you learn how to use NRTs correctly.

- The two oral medications (Zyban or Chantix) require a prescription and should be started weeks before your scheduled quit date.

- Combination therapies, including the patch and short-acting NRT or oral therapy plus NRT, are important to consider. Combinations can be more effective.

- E-cigs are poorly studied and are unregulated. New reports of vaping-associated severe lung disease and deaths make it clear they are not safe. Major medical societies do not support their use for smoking cessation, and tobacco companies are increasingly promoting them. Do not assume they are safe or effective for smoking cessation.

- Alternative therapies such as acupuncture or hypnotherapy appear to be safe, but their effectiveness is poorly understood. If you choose one or the other, combine them with proven therapies.

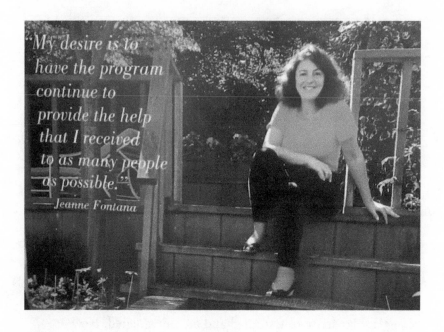

"My desire is to have the program continue to provide the help that I received to as many people as possible."
—Jeanne Fontana

Fontana Tobacco Treatment Center
1701 Divisadero St., Suite 100
San Francisco, CA 94115
Phone: (415) 885-7895

For more information, visit:

www.learningtoquit.com/fontana

This book is brought to you by the UCSF Fontana Tobacco Treatment Center.

The **UCSF Fontana Tobacco Treatment Center** offers classes as well as individual consultations with health-care professionals trained in treating tobacco addiction. We help smokers maximize the likelihood of quitting for good.

The center was named in memory of Jeanne Fontana, who was grateful to the center for helping her overcome her addiction to cigarettes. She made the Fontana Tobacco Treatment Center a beneficiary of her trust to fund current programs and establish an endowment to support future programs. The center's services include:

Stop Smoking Class

This four-week interactive course focuses on smoking and health, addiction, motivation and strategies for quitting. The class is led by Suzanne Harris, a registered nurse and certified tobacco treatment specialist; Lisa Kroon, a pharmacist and tobacco treatment specialist; and Carol Schulte, a social worker. Classes meet on Monday evenings at the Mount Zion campus and on Friday mornings at the Parnassus campus.

Freedom From Smoking Support Group

This class is for graduates of the Stop Smoking Class, including those who aren›t yet smoke-free. It provides extra support to help people become and stay smoke free.

If you enjoyed reading this book and found the information valuable, please consider leaving a review on Amazon. Your review will help other future non-smokers find the book. Thank you!

References

Preface

Jha P, Peto R: Global effects of smoking, of quitting, and of taxing tobacco. *N Engl J Med.* 2014; 370:60–68.

U.S. Surgeon General: The health consequences of smoking—50 years of progress. Atlanta, Department of Health and Human Services, 2014.

Chapter 11

Fletcher C, Peto R. The natural history of chronic airflow obstruction. *BMJ.* 1977;1:1645–1648.

Lokke A, et al: Developing COPD: A 25-year followup study of the general population. *Thorax.* 2006; 61:935–939.

Lozano R, et al.: Global and regional mortality from 235 causes of death for 20 age groups in 1990 and 2010: A systematic analysis for the Global Burden of Disease Study 2010. *Lancet.* 2012; 380:2095–2128.

National Lung Health Education Project: *www.nlhep.org*

Vestbo J, et al: Global strategy for the diagnosis, management, and prevention of chronic obstructive pulmonary disease: GOLD executive summary. *Am J Respir Crit Care Med.*2013;187:347–365.

Wheaton AG, Cunningham TJ, Ford ES, Croft JB. Employment and activity limitations among adults with chronic obstructive pulmonary disease—United States, 2013. *MMWR Morb Mortal Wkly Rep.* 2015; 64:289–95

Yang G, et. al: Rapid health transition in China, 1990-2010: Findings from the Global Burden of Disease Study 2010. *Lancet.* 2013; 381: 1987–2015.

Chapter 12

Aubin HJ, et al.: Weight gain in smokers after quitting cigarettes: Meta-analysis. *BMJ.* 2012; 345: e4439.

Chelland Campbell S, et al.: Smoking and smoking cessation—the relationship between cardiovascular disease and lipoprotein metabolism: A review. *Atherosclerosis.* 2008; 201: 225-235.

Cryer P, et al: Norepinephrine and epinephrine release and adrenergic mediation of smoking associated changes in hemodynamic and metabolic events. *N Engl J Med*. 1976; 295: 573–577.

Czernin J, Waldherr C: Cigarette smoking and coronary blood flow. Prog *Cardiovasc Dis*. 2003;45:395–404.

Gastaldelli A, et al.: Impact of tobacco smoking on lipid metabolism, body weight and cardiometabolic risk. *Curr Pharm Des*. 2010;16:2526–2530.

Godtfredsen NS, Prescott E: Benefits of smoking cessation with focus on cardiovascular and respiratory comorbidities. *Clin Respir J*. 2011;5:187–194.

Jha P, Peto R: Global effects of smoking, of quitting, and of taxing tobacco. N Engl J Med. 2014;370:60–68.

Morris PB et al.: Cardiovascular effects of exposure to cigarette smoke and electronic cigarettes: Clinical perspectives from the Prevention of Cardiovascular Disease Section Leadership Council and Early Career Councils of the American College of Cardiology. *J Am Coll Cardiol*. 2015;66:1378–1391.

Mozaffarian D, et al.: Heart disease and stroke statistics—2015 update: A report from the American Heart Association. *Circulation*. 2015;131:e29–322.

Parsons A, et al.: Influence of smoking cessation after diagnosis of early stage lung cancer on prognosis: Systematic review of observational studies with meta-analysis. *BMJ*. 2010;340:b5569.

Quillen J, et al.: Acute effect of cigarette smoking on the coronary circulation: Constriction of epicardial and resistance vessels. *J Am Coll Cardiol*. 1993; 22: 642–647.

Chapter 13

Centers for Disease Control and Prevention: Lung cancer statistics. 2018. Available online at *www.cdc.gov/cancer/lung/statistics/*.

Centers for Disease Control and Prevention: United States Cancer Statistics: Data Visualizations. 2018. Available online at *gis.cdc.gov/Cancer/USCS/DataViz.html*.

Freedman ND, et al.: Association between smoking and risk of bladder cancer among men and women; *JAMA*. 2011;306:737–745.

Hecht SS: Tobacco smoke carcinogens and lung cancer. *J Natl Cancer Inst*. 1999;91:1194–1210.

Henley SJ et al.: Lung cancer incidence trends among men and women—United States, 2005–2009. *MMWR Morb Mortal Wkly Rep.* 2014; 63:1–5.

Henley SJ, et al: Invasive cancer incidence and survival—United States, 2012. *MMWR Morb Mortal Wkly Rep.* 2015;64;1353–1358.

International Agency for Research on Cancer Working Group on the Evaluation of Carcinogenic Risks to Humans: Tobacco Smoke and Involuntary Smoking. Lyon, WHO, 2004.

Lortet-Tieulent J, et al.: State-level cancer mortality attributable to cigarette smoking in the United States. *JAMA Intern Med.* 2016;176:1792–1798.

Mukherjee S: *The Emperor of all Maladies: A Biography of Cancer.* New York, Scribner, 2010.

Murata M, et al.: A nested case-control study on alcohol drinking, tobacco smoking, and cancer. *Cancer Detect Prev.* 1996; 20: 557–565.

National Lung Screening Trial Research Team: Reduced lung-cancer mortality with low-dose computed tomographic screening. *N Engl J Med.* 2011; 365:395–409.

Osler W: *Principles and Practice of Medicine.* New York, D. Appleton and Company, 1896.

Pesch B, et al.: Cigarette smoking and lung cancer—relative risk estimates for the major histological types from a pooled analysis of case-control studies. *Int J Cancer.* 2012;131:1210–1219.

Schroeder SA: American health improvement depends upon addressing class disparities. *Prev Med.* 2016;92:6–15.

Swanton C, Govindan R: Clinical implications of genomic discoveries in lung cancer. *N Engl J Med.* 2016;374:1864–1873.

U.S. Department of Health and Human Services: *The Health Consequences of Smoking—50 Years of Progress: A Report of the Surgeon General.* 2014. Available online at *www.hhs.gov/surgeongeneral/reports-and-publications/tobacco/index.html.*

Vineis P, et al.: Tobacco and cancer: Recent epidemiological evidence. *J Natl Cancer Inst.* 2004; 96: 99–106.

Wender R et al.: American Cancer Society lung cancer screening guidelines. *CA Cancer J Clin.* 2013; 63: 107–117.

World Health Organization: Cancer. Available online at *www.who.int/mediacentre/factsheets/fs297/en/.*

Chapter 14

Benowitz N: Nicotine addiction. *N Engl J Med.* 2010; 362: 2295–2303.

Berlin I, Anthenelli RM: Monoamine oxidases and tobacco smoking. *Int J Neuropsychopharmacol.* 2001; 4: 33–42.

Brodwin E, Gal S: The 5 most addictive substances on the planet, ranked. 2016. Available online at *www.businessinsider.com/most-addictive-drugs-ranked-2016-10.*

Hasin DS, et al.: Epidemiology of adult DSM-5 major depressive disorder and its specifiers in the United States. *JAMA Psychiatry.* 2018; 75: 336–346.

Hogg RC: Contribution of monoamine oxidase inhibition to tobacco dependence: A review of the evidence. *Nicotine Tob Res.* 2016; 18: 509–523.

Hughes JR: Clinical significance of tobacco withdrawal. *Nicotine Tob Res.* 2006; 8: 153–156.

Jones R, et al: Therapeutics for Nicotine Addiction, in

Neuropsychopharmacology: The Fifth Generation of Progress. Davis KL, et al. (eds.). Philadelphia, Lippincott Williams & Wilkins, 2002.

Kotz D, et al.: Prospective cohort study of the effectiveness of smoking cessation treatments used in the "real world." *Mayo Clin Proc.* 2014; 89: 1360–1367.

Nutt D, et al.: Development of a rational scale to assess the harm of drugs of potential misuse. *Lancet.* 2007; 369:1047–1053.

Perry DC, et al.: Increased nicotinic receptors in brains from smokers: Membrane binding and autoradiography studies. *J Pharmacol Exp Ther.* 1999; 289: 1545–1552.

Simpson T: Indian tobacco: The non-abusive use of tobacco by Native Americans. 2008. Available online at *www.stogiefresh.info/edu-health/articles/indian-tobacco.html.*

Stepankova L, et al.: Depression and smoking cessation: Evidence from a smoking cessation clinic with 1-year follow-up. *Ann Behav Med.* 2017; 51: 454–463.

van Amsterdam J, et al.: Ranking the harm of alcohol, tobacco and illicit drugs for the individual and the population. *Eur Addict Res.* 2010;16:202–207.

Chapter 15

Ahluwalia JS, et al.: Sustained-release bupropion for smoking cessation in African Americans: A randomized controlled trial. *JAMA.* 2002; 288: 468–474.

Alzahrani T,Pena I,Temesgen N,Glantz SA Association Between Electronic Cigarette Use and Myocardial Infarction. *Am Jnl Prev Med.* 2018 Oct; 55(4): 455-461;

American College of Obstetricians and Gynecologists: Smoking cessation during pregnancy. Committee opinion no. 471. *Obstet Gynecol.* 2010; 116: 1241–1244.

Anthenelli RM, et al.: Neuropsychiatric safety and efficacy of varenicline, bupropion, and nicotine patch in smokers with and without psychiatric disorders (EAGLES): A double-blind, randomized, placebo-controlled clinical trial. *Lancet.* 2016; 387: 2507–2520.

Barrington-Trimis, JL, Leventhal, AM; Adolescents' Use of "Pod Mod" E-Cigarettes – Urgent Concerns; New 2018 Sep 20;379(12):1099-1102.

Benowitz NL, Brunetta PG: Smoking Hazards and Cessation, in Murray and Nadel's *Textbook of Respiratory Medicine,* 6th ed. Philadelphia, Saunders, 2016.

Bérard A, et al.: Success of smoking cessation interventions during pregnancy. *Am J Obstet Gynecol.* 2016; 215: 611.

Borrelli B, O'Connor GT, *New England Journal of Medicine;* 2019 Feb 14; 380(7): 678-679;2019 Jan 30. E-Cigarettes to Assist with Smoking Cessation.

Cahill K, et al.: Pharmacological interventions for smoking cessation: An overview and network meta-analysis. *Cochrane Database Syst Rev.* 2013; 5: CD009329.

Centers for Disease Control and Prevention: Quitting smoking among adults—United States. 2001–2010. *MMWR Morb Mortal Wkly Rep.* 2011; 60:1513–1519.

Centers for Disease Control and Prevention: Severe Lung Disease. Available online at *www.cdc.gov/tobacco/basic_information/e-cigarettes/severe-lung-disease.html#latest-outbreak-information*

Centers for Disease Control and Prevention: Tobacco use in pregnancy. Available online at *www.cdc.gov/reproductivehealth/maternalinfanthealth/tobaccousepregnancy/.*

Chaffee BW, Watkins SL, Glantz SA; Electronic Cigarette Use and Progression From Experimentation to Established Smoking; *Pediatrics.* 2018 Apr;141(4).

Chamberlain C, et al.: Psychosocial interventions for supporting women to stop smoking in pregnancy. *Cochrane Database Sys Rev.* 2013;10:CD001055.

Chantix [package insert]. New York, Pfizer Labs, 2014.

Choi JH, et al.: Pharmacokinetics of a nicotine polacrilex lozenge. *Nicotine Tob Res.* 2003; 5: 635–644.

Coe JW, et al.: Varenicline: An $\alpha_4\beta_2$ nicotinic receptor partial agonist for smoking cessation. *J Med Chem.* 2005; 48: 3474–3477.

Coleman T, et al.: A randomized trial of nicotine-replacement therapy patches in pregnancy. *N Engl J Med.* 2012; 366: 808–818.

Cooper S, et al.: Smoking, Nicotine and Pregnancy (SNAP) Trial Team. Effect of nicotine patches in pregnancy on infant and maternal outcomes at 2 years: Follow-up from the randomized, double-blind, placebo-controlled SNAP trial. *Lancet Respir Med.* 2014; 2: 728–737.

Corelli RL, Hudmon KS: Pharmacologic interventions for smoking cessation. *Crit Care Nurs Clin North Am.* 2006;18: 39–51.

Crowley RA: Electronic nicotine delivery systems: Executive summary of a policy position paper from the American College of Physicians. *Ann Intern Med.* 2015; 162: 583–584.

Cryan JF, et al.: Non-nicotinic neuropharmacological strategies for nicotine dependence: Beyond bupropion. *Drug Discov Today.* 2003; 8:1025–1034.

Davidson K. Brancato A, Heetderks P, Mansour W, Matheis E, Nario M, Rajagopalan S, Underhill B, Wininger J, Fox D; Outbreak of Electronic-Cigarette-Associated Acute Lipoid Pneumonia – North Carolina, July-August 2019. *MMWR Morb Mortal Wkly Report.* 2019, Sep 13; 68(36):784-786

Ebbert JO, et al.: Combination pharmacotherapy for stopping smoking: What advantages does it offer? *Drugs.* 2010;70:643–650.

Ebbert JO, et al.: Combination varenicline and bupropion SR for tobacco-dependence treatment in cigarette smokers: A randomized trial. JAMA. 2014; 311:155–163.

Ebbert JO, et al.: Effect of varenicline on smoking cessation through smoking reduction: A randomized clinical trial. *JAMA.* 2015; 313: 687–694.

Els C, et al.: Smoking cessation and neuropsychiatric adverse events. *Can Fam Physician.* 2011; 57: 647–649.

Fiore M, et al.: Tobacco use and dependence guideline panel. *Treating tobacco use and dependence: 2008 update.* Rockville, MD, U.S. Department of Health and Human Services, 2008.

Gonzales D, et al.: Retreatment with varenicline for smoking cessation in smokers who have previously taken varenicline: A randomized, placebo-controlled trial. *Clin Pharmacol Ther.* 2014;.96:390–396.

Hajek P, et al.: Use of varenicline for 4 weeks before quitting smoking: Decrease in ad lib smoking and increase in smoking cessation rates. *Arch Intern Med.* 2011;171:770–777.

Hajek P, Phillips-Waller A, Przuli D, Pesola F, Myers Smith K, Bisal N, Li J, Parrott S, Sasieni P, Dawkins L, Ross L, Goniewicz M, Wu Q, McRobbie HJ; *New England Journal of Medicine.* 2019. Feb 14; 380(7): 629-637. Jan 30.A Randomized Trial of E-Cigarettes versus Nicotine-Replacement Therapy.

Hall SM, et al.: Psychological intervention and antidepressant treatment in smoking cessation. *Arch Gen Psychiatry.* 2002; 59:930–936.

Hawkes N: E-cigarettes may work as well as nicotine patches in reducing and quitting smoking, but evidence is limited. *BMJ.* 2014; 349: g7722.

Hsia SL, et al.: Combination nicotine replacement therapy: Strategies for initiation and tapering. *Prev Med.* 2017; 97: 45–49.

https://www.cdc.gov/media/releases/2019/s0912-update-cases-vaping.html

Hughes JR, et al.: Antidepressants for smoking cessation. *Cochrane Database Syst Rev.* 2014;1:CD000031.

Jorenby DE, et al.: Comparative efficacy and tolerability of nicotine replacement therapies. *CNS Drugs.* 1995; 3: 227–236.

Kralikova E, et al.: Fifty-two-week continuous abstinence rates of smokers being treated with varenicline versus nicotine replacement therapy. *Addiction.* 2013; 108: 1497–1502.

Koegelenberg CF, et al.: Efficacy of varenicline combined with nicotine replacement therapy vs varenicline alone for smoking cessation: A randomized clinical trial. JAMA. 2014; 312: 155–156.

Layden JE, Ghinai I, Pray I, Kimball A, Layer M, Tenforde M,Navon L, Hoots B, Salvatore PP, Elderbrook M, Haupt T, Kanne J,Patel MT, Saathoff-Huber L, King BA, Schier JG, Mikosz CA, Meiman J. *New England Journal of Medicine.*2019 Sep 6;Pulmonary Illness Related to E-Cigarette Use in Illinois and Wisconsin – Preliminary Report.

Le Houezec J: Role of nicotine pharmacokinetics in nicotine addiction and nicotine replacement therapy: A review. Int J *Tuberc Lung Dis.* 2003;7: 811–819.

Malas M, et al.: Electronic cigarettes for smoking cessation: A systematic review. *Nicotine Tob Res.* 2016; 18: 1926–1936.

Malarcher A, et al.: Quitting smoking among adults—United States, 2001–2010. *MMWR Morb Mortal Wkly Rep.* 2011; 60: 1513–1519.

McRobbie H, et al.: Electronic cigarettes for smoking cessation and reduction. *Cochrane Database Syst Rev.* 2014;12:CD010216.

Miech R, Johnston L, O'Malley PM, Bachman JG, Patrick ME; Trends in Adolescent Vaping, 2017-2019; New England Journal of Medicine 2019, Oct 10;381(15):1490-1491

Mills EJ, et al.: Cardiovascular events associated with smoking cessation pharmacotherapies: A network meta-analysis. *Circulation.* 2014; 129: 28–41.

Mitchell JM, et al.: Varenicline decreases alcohol consumption in heavy-drinking smokers. *Psychopharmacology* (Berl). 2012; 223: 299–306.

Moore TJ, et al.: Suicidal behavior and depression in smoking cessation treatments. *PLoS One.* 2011; 6: e27016.

Morris PB, et al.: Cardiovascular effects of exposure to cigarette smoke and electronic cigarettes: Clinical perspectives from the Prevention of Cardiovascular Disease Section Leadership Council and Early Career Councils of the American College of Cardiology. *J Am Coll Cardiol.* 2015; 66: 1378–1391.

National Academies of Sciences, Engineering, and Medicine: Public Health Consequences of E-Cigarettes. Washington, DC, National Academies Press, 2018. Available online at *www.nap.edu/read/24952/chapter/1.*

Nicorette® Gum [package insert]. Moon Township, PA, GlaxoSmithKline Consumer Healthcare, 2014.

Nicorette® Lozenge [package insert]. Moon Township, PA, GlaxoSmithKline Consumer Healthcare, 2015.

NicoDerm® CQ [package insert]. Moon Township, PA, GlaxoSmithKline Consumer Healthcare, 2015.

Nicotrol® Inhaler [package insert]. New York, Pharmacia and Upjohn, 2008.

Nicotrol® NS [package insert]. New York, Pharmacia and Upjohn, 2010.

Rahman MA, Hann N, Wilson A, Mnatzaganian G, Worrall-Carter L; *PLos One.* 2015 Mar 30; 10(3); E-cigarettes and smoking cessation: evidence from a systematic review and meta-analysis.

Ramon JM, et al.: Combining varenicline and nicotine patches: A randomized controlled trial study in smoking cessation. *BMC Med.* 2014; 12: 172.

Romagna G, et al.: Cytotoxicity evaluation of electronic cigarette vapor extract on cultured mammalian fibroblasts (ClearStream-LIFE): Comparison with tobacco cigarette smoke extract. *Inhal Toxicol.* 2013; 25: 354–361.

Rose JE, Behm FM: Combination treatment with varenicline and bupropion in an adaptive smoking cessation paradigm. *Am J Psychiatry.* 2014; 171: 1199–1205.

Schneider NG, et al.: The nicotine inhaler: Clinical pharmacokinetics and comparison with other nicotine treatments. *Clin Pharmacokinet.* 2001; 40: 661–684.

Schnoll RA, et al.: High dose transdermal nicotine for fast metabolizers of nicotine: A proof of concept placebo-controlled trial. *Nicotine Tob Res.* 2013;15: 348–354.

Siu AL: Behavioral and pharmacotherapy interventions for tobacco smoking cessation in adults, including pregnant women: U.S. Preventive Services Task Force recommendation statement. *Ann Intern Med.* 2015; 163: 622–634.

Sommerfeld CG, et al.: Hypersensitivity pneumonitis and acute respiratory distress syndrome from e-cigarette use. *Pediatrics.* 2018; 141: e20163927.

Soneji S, et al.: Association between initial use of e-cigarettes and subsequent cigarette smoking among adolescents and young adults: A systematic review and meta-analysis. *JAMA Pediatr.* 2017; 171: 788–797.

Stead LF, et al.: Nicotine replacement therapy for smoking cessation. *Cochrane Database Syst Rev.* 2012; 11: CD000146.

Thomas KH, et al.: Risk of neuropsychiatric adverse events associated with varenicline: Systematic review and meta-analysis. *BMJ.* 2015; 350: h1109.

Thomas KH, et al.: Smoking cessation treatment and risk of depression, suicide, and self-harm in the clinical practice research datalink: Prospective cohort study. *BMJ.* 2013; 347: f5704.

Tolentino J: Vaping and the rise of Juul. *The New Yorker.* May 14, 2018.

Verbiest M, et al.: National guidelines for smoking cessation in primary care: A literature review and evidence analysis. *NPJ Prim Care Respir Med.* 2017; 27: 2.

Warner C, Shoaib M: How does bupropion work as a smoking cessation aid? *Addict Biol.* 2005; 10: 23–35.

Wightman DS, et al.: Meta-analysis of suicidality in placebo-controlled clinical trials of adults taking bupropion. *Prim Care Companion J Clin Psychiatry.* 2010; 12:5.

Zyban [package insert]. Research Park Triangle, NC, GlaxoSmithKline, 2015.

Acknowledgments

Special Thanks from Suzanne Harris

This book would not exist were it not for **Trisha Winder Clevenger**. As the enlightened Nurse Manager of the SFGH Adult Medical General Medical Clinic, she gave her nursing staff the option to develop programs for issues for which we had a special interest and passion. Recognizing that many of our patients had medical conditions that were worsened, if not caused, by smoking, I elected to address the need for cessation support and treatment. It was from that early beginning in 1984 that this book eventually began to take shape.

Every life brings remarkable characters that shape a personal and professional destiny. **Clarence Brown** is such a character in mine. Witnessing, and being a part of his transformation from a grumpy, cantankerous, difficult smoker into a regal and charismatic smoke-free community leader, brought me lessons and gifts. Clarence showed me that even for people who have become seriously ill from smoking, quitting changes life for the better. He modeled what a difference stopping smoking can make in how people feel about themselves and how they move in the world.

It was Clarence who inadvertently led me to know **John Harding**. Through a member of Group (Barbara Vos), John volunteered to do a portrait of one of our members for a publicity poster. John was so taken with his experience of photographing Clarence, he suggested that he and I embark on a project to document the stories of more participants, thus leading to the collection of images and interviews that have become *Learning to Quit*. Through John, I was given the inspiring opportunity to travel around San Francisco and be welcomed into the homes of people I'd only known in the context of the hospital. My debt to John Harding is immeasurable.

Of course, the next stage of evolution to this book would never have happened without the enthusiastic endorsement of my dear friend, **Paul Brunetta**. When I showed Paul a handful of photocopied interviews and portraits, he insisted that what I was holding was the beginning of a book that could help people beyond the immediate touch of our groups and clinic visits. It took some persuading, but the idea took root and the rest is history.

How we converse with one another and ourselves has everything to do with personal change and quality of life. Being able to communicate with compassion and without judgment can be critical. Motivational Interviewing is based on these values, and I have been blessed with a master teacher, **Sheila Stevens**, from the Mayo Clinic. I can think of no one who surpasses her skill; and her influence on my work is immeasurable.

Some of us are fortunate to have children who become our teachers. One example is my daughter, **Jenny Bender**. An early reader of this book and a published author herself, Jenny gave us insight that has been instrumental in focusing the stories and text. In addition, her support and encouragement have been unfailing, and her willingness to add her own story to this collection only deepens my gratitude.

Thank you to **Penny Wisner** who persuaded me that I had something to say and could find a way to say it. And then to **Mary McKenney** who took up that cry and added her expert editing skills to the early chapters. **Sharon Silva**, editor extraordinaire, has left her indelible and professional mark on this project as well. **Nancy Ippolito** and **Cecilia Brunazzi** have been generous with their time and skills in publishing and graphic design. My sister **Christine Charest** gave feedback on early versions of this book.

Linda John has been an unrelenting supporter for its completion.

At UCSF, I am fortunate to enjoy the support and partnership of a remarkable group of people dedicated to serving the needs of patients who smoke. First in this group is my dear friend and co-director of the Fontana Tobacco Treatment Center (FTTC), **Lisa Kroon**. Lisa generously offers her brilliance to the group program, giving a lesson on all the current medications available to treat withdrawal symptoms while one is becoming a non-smoker. She is an invaluable partner in directing the development and services of the FTTC. I am most fortunate to have her trustworthy guidance and leadership. **Joan Schoonover** has shared this work with me for the duration of our friendship. Our many conversations about each another's work have added quality and depth to my own.

Joanna DeLong, **Michele Francis**, and **Karen Rago** have provided invaluable support as managers over the years. In addition, significant leaders in the effort to secure quality tobacco treatment also have contributed to the development of the FTTC: **Gina Intinarelli**, **Neal Benowitz**, **Steve Schroeder**, **Stan Glantz**, **Radhika Ramanan**, and **Carol Schulte**. **Ernie Rosenbaum** was an early supporter and secured funding for what eventually became the FTTC. **David Claman** recognized the importance of helping smokers learn how to stop and generously provided space for us in his Pulmonary Clinic.

The continued existence of the FTTC is due to the immensely generous contribution of **Jeanne Fontana**. We strive to be guided by the intent of her bequest, that "as many people as possible receive the services and support to become smoke free that she did." There are many whose lives have been saved by her gift, and there will be many more.

All through this project, both the book and the program, there have been dozens of people who donated their time and expertise because they recognized the importance of supporting people to stop smoking. **Dianne Derby** was one of these people who had an especially powerful contribution to make to the program itself.

Finally: Over the years, there have been many friends and supporters who have generously given their time and encouragement to this book. While unnamed, they are nonetheless critical to its creation.

Special Thanks from Paul Brunetta

I'm most grateful for the inspiration I've gained from **Suzanne** over the many years we've worked together. She's been a constant source of exceptional counseling for people with nicotine addiction and has a unique empathy and understanding. Without her, this project never would have begun. Along the way we gained initial support from the Mount Zion Health Fund and **Ernie Rosenbaum**, who connected us to the fund. Ernie was a much beloved oncologist at Mount Zion Hospital with a desire to do anything that could prevent the cancers he treated in so many patients. As we expanded the program, **Lisa Kroon**, now the Chair of Clinical Pharmacology at UCSF, joined the program and became a constant guiding presence and ardent supporter of the group counseling program. Along the way, she and **Robin Corelli** and **Karen Hudmon** developed a tremendous educational resource called RxforChange that explains smoking cessation medications to health-care providers. Of course, without the tremendous generosity of **Jeannie Fontana**, we couldn't have realized the long-term viability of the Fontana Tobacco Treatment Center. Jeannie's stated desire before she died was "to have the program continue to provide the help that I received to as many people as possible." FTTC is dedicated to this mission, and this book is part of it—a percentage of the proceeds will be returned to FTTC to support expansion.

Several faculty members are a special inspiration for this book. **Neal Benowitz** is a tremendous physician and international expert on nicotine and has contributed to many Surgeon General reports along with hundreds of articles in the field. His dedication over several decades is a guiding light for us. **Stan Glantz** is a central figure in the UCSF Center for Tobacco Control Research and

Education and author of The Cigarette Papers and Tobacco War, and has influenced smoking policy around the world and prevented countless—literally millions—of deaths. UCSF is a treasure trove of young researchers mining the internal tobacco company documents and working to bring balance to the injustice of nicotine addiction. The annual Billion Lives Symposium, named after the number of people expected to die this 21st century from tobacco-related disease, is a major inspiration and source of information.

I'd like to thank my wonderful partner, **Ann**, for her support over the many years, along with my twins, **Taite** and **Sam**, for their interest in this book and feedback on my lectures about smoking to their middle and high schools. My friend **Brian Spahr** quit smoking and early on helped me realize what messages might help someone along his or her path to committing to better health. And my sister, **Lisa Carano**, has always been a source of unconditional love (and great cookies) and inspired me to keep working on *Learning to Quit*.

And most recently, this book might never have been realized without a connection to an immensely talented editor and guide, **Greg Feldman**. **Dawn Repola** helped us find Greg, who then brought in **Nicole French** for editing and **Kelsey Martin** for design and layout or our first released version. Most recently, **Deirdre Kennedy** helped Suzanne and I find **Kelsye Nelson** at Avasta Press, who's been instrumental in this revision of *Learning to Quit*. Figure illustration was beautifully provided and updated by **Tess Marhofer**. As we look back, it's taken more than a decade and thousands of hours to craft a book designed to impact behavioral change, and many individuals have played a critical role in completing our vision. We hope this book helps the reader turn thought into action.

Would you like to use *Learning to Quit* as a resource to support your smoking cessation group, patients or organization? Special discounts are available on quantity purchases. Please visit www.learningtoquit.com/order for more information.

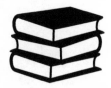

Would you like to use Learning to Quit as a resource to support your smoking cessation group, patients or organization? Special discounts are available on quantity purchases.

www.learningtoquit.com/order

CPSIA information can be obtained
at www.ICGtesting.com
Printed in the USA
LVHW011519060521
686701LV00001B/96